LOVE YOURSELF WITH DASH DIET

Love your Heart and Lower Blood Pressure and Cholesterol. The Complete Dash Diet Recipe Book to Improve your Health!

ELEANOR FIELDS

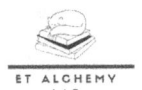

ET ALCHEMY LAB

CONTENTS

Introduction	v
1. Why Dash Diet?	1
2. Breakfast	4
3. Lunch	16
4. Dinner	72
5. Snacks & Desserts	97
6. Conclusions	116

© Copyright 2021 - Eleanor Fields - All rights reserved.

The content contained within this book may not be reproduced, duplicated or transmitted without direct written permission from the author or the publisher.

Under no circumstances will any blame or legal responsibility be held against the publisher, or author, for any damages, reparation, or monetary loss due to the information contained within this book. Either directly or indirectly.

Legal Notice:

This book is copyright protected. This book is only for personal use. You cannot amend, distribute, sell, use, quote or paraphrase any part, or the content within this book, without the consent of the author or publisher.

Disclaimer Notice:

Please note the information contained within this document is for educational and entertainment purposes only. All effort has been executed to present accurate, up to date, and reliable, complete information. No warranties of any kind are declared or implied. Readers acknowledge that the author is not engaging in the rendering of legal, financial, medical or professional advice. The content within this book has been derived from various sources. Please consult a licensed professional before attempting any techniques outlined in this book.

By reading this document, the reader agrees that under no circumstances is the author responsible for any losses, direct or indirect, which are incurred as a result of the use of information contained within this document, including, but not limited to, — errors, omissions, or inaccuracies.

INTRODUCTION

The past two decades have seen a sudden increase in the number of people with high blood pressure. People with high blood pressure has increased in the last years. With so many people unable to control their blood pressure, it's safe to say that our millennial lifestyle has played a significant role in producing this troubling result.

To counter this, the U.S. Department of Health and Human Services has promoted the DASH diet, an effective way to combat hypertension among people. The diet results from scientists' careful study of various foods that help people control rising blood pressure levels.

The recipes mentioned in the book will help you stay on track with a healthy lifestyle. Not only will you witness a gradual drop in blood pressure, but you can also enjoy the process by creating recipes that are easy to cook and taste great.

The book has a detailed 21-day plan that includes recipes for breakfast, lunch, and dinner. With the help of this guide, you will never be left out due to increased blood pressure. Enjoy the recipes and do most of the healthy eating. With this book by your side, no day will ever be dull. Eat healthily, stay healthy.

Chapter One
WHY DASH DIET?

According to the dash diet plan, you need about four servings of vegetables, four servings of fruits, and 2-3 servings of low-fat dairy products. If you compare these portions with those of the average American's diet, you will see that the latter contains only one or less serving of dairy products and 3-4 servings of fruits and vegetables. You should also consume poultry, fish, and nuts. You need to limit red meat, sugary foods, drinks, and fatty foods for these nutritious foods.

Eat this balanced diet of nutritious and healthy foods for 14 days, and you will see noticeable differences in your blood pressure readings and overall health. If your blood pressure is "slightly" high, it will decrease to a level where your doctor may recommend you stop taking medication. Stick to the Dash diet to take advantage of key other mental and physical health benefits.

Dash in simple steps

Figuring out how to implement the dash plan is as simple as three easy steps. So, let's get started.

Step 1 - Determine your caloric goal.

Every individual has different energy needs. For example, the energy needs of a 130-pound senior citizen are other than those of a 170-pound football player.

When practicing dash, you should take the first step to determine the number of calories you should take each day. Once easily calculated online, you can decide which type of diet for dash you should consume.

Step 2 - Identify the ideal dash diet for your calorie goal

You already know your required calorie intake, as you now determine which dash diet can give you efficient results. This will further help you decide how many servings you need from each food group to stay healthy and active.

Step 3 - Ready for the Dash

The following steps are as necessary as controlling high blood pressure to use the dash the right way.

- Discuss your eating plan with your doctor and have him or her analyze your blood pressure readings.

- Mark the day you plan to start the dash eating plan on your calendar.

- Inform friends and family that you are practicing the hyphen diet, as they can support you in your efforts.

- Get rid of all food items that are not part of the hyphen food plan, especially chips, candy bars, ice cream, and other snacks.

- Change your habits. Don't eat in front of the television. Get physical activity as part of your daily routine.

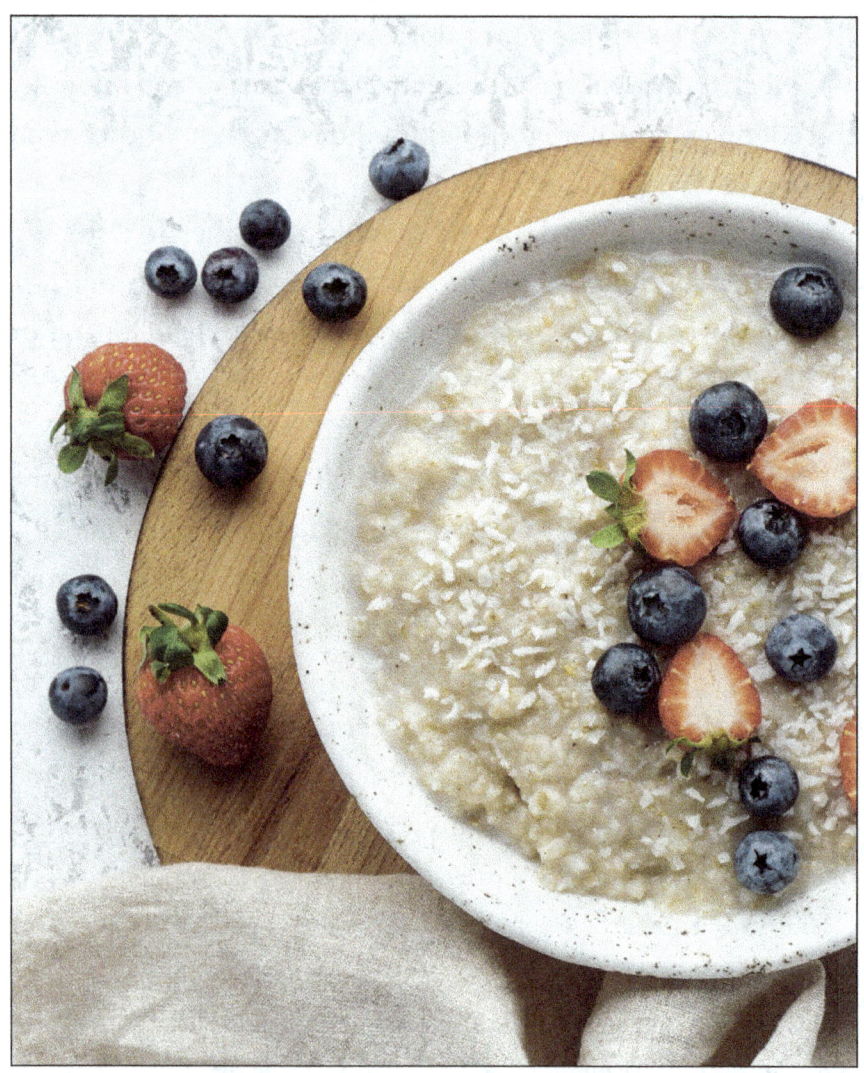

Chapter Two

BREAKFAST

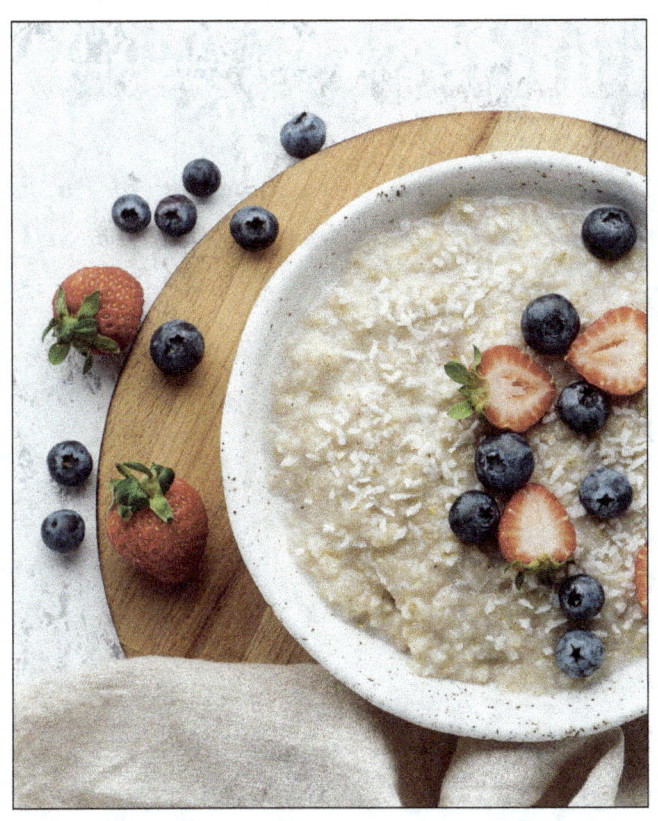

BANANA STEEL OATS

Preparation time: *10 min*
Cooking time: *15 min*
Portions: 3
Ingredients:
1 small banana
1 cup of almond milk
¼ tsp cinnamon, ground
Ingredients:
½ cup rolled oats
1 tbsp honey
Directions:
Take a saucepan and add half the banana, whisk in almond milk, ground cinnamon.
Season with the sunflower seeds. Stir until the banana is well mashed, bring the mixture to the boil and stir in the oats.
Reduce the heat to medium-low and simmer for 5-7 min until the oats are tender.
Dice the remaining half of the banana and place it on top of the oatmeal. Enjoy your meal!
Preparation time: *10 min*
Cooking time: *4-8 hours*
Portions: 5
Ingredients:
1 cup steel-cut oats
4 cups unsweetened almond milk

2 medium-sized apples, sliced

1 tsp of coconut oil

Ingredients:

1 tsp cinnamon

¼ tsp nutmeg

2 tbsps maple syrup, unsweetened

A trickle of lemon juice

Directions:

Add the listed ingredients to a saucepan and mix well. Cook on a very low heat for 8 hours or on a high heat for 4 hours.

Stir gently. Add the desired toppings. Serve and enjoy!

Store in the fridge for later use; be sure to add a splash of almond milk after heating to add flavour.

CRISPY FLAX AND ALMOND CRACKERS

Preparation time: 15 min
Cooking time: 60 min
Servings size: 20-24 crackers
Ingredients:
½ cup ground linseed
½ cup of almond flour
1 tbsp of coconut flour
2 tbsps shelled hemp seeds
Ingredients:
¼ tsp of sunflower seeds
1 egg white

2 tbsps unsalted almond butter, melted

Directions:

Preheat the oven to 300 degrees F.

Line a baking tray with baking paper, set aside.

Add the flax, almonds, coconut flour and hemp seeds to a bowl and mix.

Add the egg whites and melted almond butter, stir until combined.

Transfer the dough onto a sheet of parchment paper and cover with another sheet of paper.

Roll out the dough. Cut into crackers and bake for 60 min. Let them cool and enjoy!

COOL MUSHROOM MUNCHIES

Preparation time: 5 min
Cooking time: 10 min
Portions: 2

Ingredients:

4 caps Portobello mushrooms

3 tbsps of coconut amino acids

2 tbsps of sesame oil

Ingredients:

1 tbsp fresh ginger, chopped

1 small clove of garlic, minced

Directions:

Set the oven to minimum, keeping the rack 15 cm from the heat source.

Wash the mushrooms under cold water and transfer them to a baking tray (top side down).
Take a bowl and mix the sesame oil, garlic, coconut amino acid, ginger and pour the mixture over the tops of the mushrooms.
Cook for 10 min. Serve and enjoy!

DELICIOUS QUINOA BOWL WITH BERRIES

Preparation time: *5 min*
Cooking time: *15 min*
Portions: *4*
Ingredients:
1 cup quinoa
2 cups of water
1 2-inch piece of cinnamon stick
2-3 tbsps of maple syrup Flavourful toppings
½ cup of blueberries, raspberries or strawberries
Ingredients:
2 tbsps of sultanas
1 tsp lime
¼ tsp nutmeg, grated
3 tbsps whipped coconut cream
2 tbsps cashews, chopped
Directions:
Take a metal strainer and pass your grains through it to filter them well.
Rinse the grains well under cold water.

Take a medium-sized saucepan and pour in the water.
Add the strained grains and bring to the boil.
Add the cinnamon sticks and cover the saucepan.
Lower the heat and let the mixture simmer for 15 min to allow the grains to absorb the liquid.
Remove from the heat and stir the mixture with a fork.
Add maple syrup if you want extra flavour.
Also, if you want to make things a little more interesting, just add any of the above ingredients.

BOWL OF QUINOA AND CINNAMON

Preparation time: 10 min
Cooking time: 15 min
Portions: 2
Ingredients:
1 cup uncooked quinoa
1½ cups of water
½ tsp cinnamon powder
Ingredients:
½ tsp of sunflower seeds
A drizzle of almond/coconut milk to serve
Directions:
Rinse the quinoa well under water.
Take a medium-sized saucepan and add the quinoa, water, cinnamon and seeds.

Stir and place over medium-high heat. Bring the mixture to the boil.

Reduce the heat to low and simmer for 10 min.

Once cooked, remove from the heat and allow to cool.

Serve with a drizzle of almond or coconut milk.

Enjoy your meal!

INCREDIBLE, HEALTHY BOWL OF GRANOLA

Preparation time: *5 min*
Cooking time: *25 min*
Portions: 6
Ingredients:
1 ounce oatmeal Porridge
2 tsp maple syrup Cooking spray if necessary
4 medium bananas
4 jars of Fromage Frais layered caramel
5 ounces of fresh fruit salad, such as strawberries, blueberries and raspberries
Ingredients:
¼ ounce pumpkin seeds
¼ ounce sunflower seeds
¼ ounce of dried chia seeds
¼ ounce of dried coconut
Directions:
Preheat the oven to 300 degrees F.
Take a baking tray and line it with baking paper.

Take a large bowl and add the oats, maple syrup and seeds.

Spread the mixture on a baking tray.

Pour the coconut oil over the top and bake for 20 min, making sure to keep stirring from time to time.

Sprinkle with coconut after the first 15 min. Remove from the oven and leave to cool.

Take a bowl and layer sliced bananas on top of the Fromage Fraise.

Spread the cooled granola mix on top and serve with a berry garnish. Enjoy!

BOWL OF QUINOA AND DATES

Preparation time: 10 min
Cooking time: 15 min
Portions: 2
Ingredients:
1 date, pitted and finely chopped
½ cup red quinoa, dried
1 cup unsweetened almond milk
Ingredients:
1/8 tsp vanilla extract
¼ cup fresh strawberries, hulled and sliced
1/8 tsp cinnamon powder
Directions:
Take a frying pan and put it on a low heat.

Add the quinoa, almond milk, cinnamon and vanilla
and cook for about 15 min,
Making sure to keep stirring from time to time.
Garnish with strawberries and enjoy!

PUMPKIN OATS

Preparation time: 5 min
Cooking time: 8 min
Portions: 3
Ingredients:
1 cup quick-cooking rolled oats
¾ cup of almond milk
½ cup canned pumpkin puree
Ingredients:
¼ tsp of pumpkin spice
1 tsp cinnamon powder
Directions:
Take a microwave-safe bowl and add the oats and
almond milk and microwave for 1-2 min.
Add more almond milk if necessary to reach the
desired consistency.
Cook for a further 30 seconds.
Stir in the pumpkin puree, pumpkin pie spice and
ground cinnamon. Heat gently and enjoy!

ENERGY-RICH OATMEAL

Preparation time: 10-15 min
Cooking time: 5 min
Portions: 2
Ingredients:
¼ cup quick-cooking oats
¼ cup of almond milk
2 tbsps low-fat Greek yoghurt
Ingredients:
¼ cup banana, mashed
2-1/4 tbsps of linseed meal
Directions:
Beat all the ingredients in a bowl.
Transfer the bowl to the refrigerator and leave to stand for 15 min.
Serve and enjoy!

MOUTH-WATERING CHICKEN PORRIDGE

Preparation time: 1 hour
Cooking time: 10-20 min
Portions: 4
Ingredients:
1 cup jasmine rice
1 pound of steamed/cooked chicken thighs
5 cups of chicken broth

Ingredients:
4 cups of water
1 ½ cups fresh ginger Green onions Roasted cashews
Directions:
Put the rice in the fridge and leave it to cool for 1 hour before cooking.
Remove the rice and add it to your Robot.
Pour in the chicken stock and water.
Close the lid and cook in PORRIDGE mode, using the default settings and parameters.
Release the pressure naturally in 10 min.
Open the lid. Remove the meat from the chicken legs and add the meat to the soup.
Stir well in Sauté mode. Season with a little aromatic vinegar and enjoy with a garnish of walnuts and onion.

THE DECISIVE APPLE 'PORRIDGE

Preparation time: 10 min
Cooking time: 5 min
Portions: 2
Ingredients:
1 large apple, peeled, stoned and grated
1 cup unsweetened almond milk
1 ½ tbsps of sunflower seeds
Ingredients:
1/8 cup fresh blueberries

¼ tsp fresh vanilla pod extract

Directions:

Take a large pan and add the sunflower seeds, vanilla extract, almond milk, apples and stir.

Place over medium-low heat. Cook for 5 min, making sure to keep the mixture stirred. Transfer to a serving bowl. Serve and enjoy

Chapter Three

LUNCH

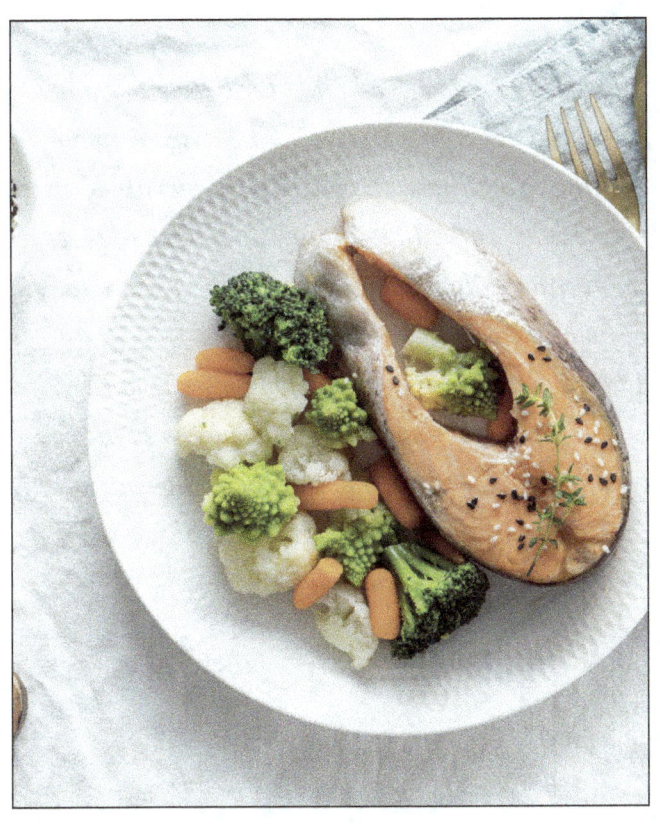

FANTASTIC MANGO CHICKEN

Preparation time: 25 min
Cooking time: 10 min
Portions: 4

Ingredients:

2 medium mangoes, peeled and cut 10 ounces of coconut milk 4 tsp of vegetable oil 4 tsp of spicy curry paste 14 ounces of boneless meat

Ingredients:

skinless chicken breast, diced 4 medium shallots 1 large English cucumber, sliced and seeded

Directions:

Slice half the mangoes and add the halves to a bowl. Add the mangoes and the almond and coconut milk to a blender and blend until smooth. Keep the mixture aside. Take a large saucepan and place it over a medium heat, add the oil and allow the oil to heat up.

Add the curry paste and cook for 1 minute until fragrant, add the shallots and chicken to the pot and cook for 5 min. Pour in the mango puree and let it warm up. Serve the cooked chicken with the mango puree and cucumbers. Enjoy

CHICKEN LIVER STEW

Preparation time: 10 min
Cooking time: Zero
Portions: 2
Ingredients:
10 ounces of chicken livers
1 ounce onion, chopped
Ingredients:
2 ounces of sour cream
1 tbsp olive oil Sunflower seeds as desired
Directions:
Take a frying pan and place it over medium heat.
Add the oil and let it warm up.
Add the onions and fry until just golden. Add the livers and season with sunflower seeds.
Cook until the livers are half cooked.
Transfer the mixture to a stew pot.
Add the sour cream and cook for 20 min. Serve and enjoy!

CHICKEN WITH MUSTARD

Preparation time: 10 min
Cooking time: 40 min
Portions: 2
Ingredients:

2 chicken breasts

1/4 cup of chicken broth

2 tbsps mustard

1 1/2 tbsps of olive oil

Ingredients:

1/2 tsp of paprika

1/2 tsp of chilli powder

1/2 tsp of garlic powder

Directions:

Take a small bowl and mix the mustard, olive oil, paprika, chicken broth, garlic powder and chilli. Add the chicken breast and marinate for 30 min. Take a lined baking tray and place the chicken on it. Bake for 35 min at 375 degrees F. Serve and enjoy!

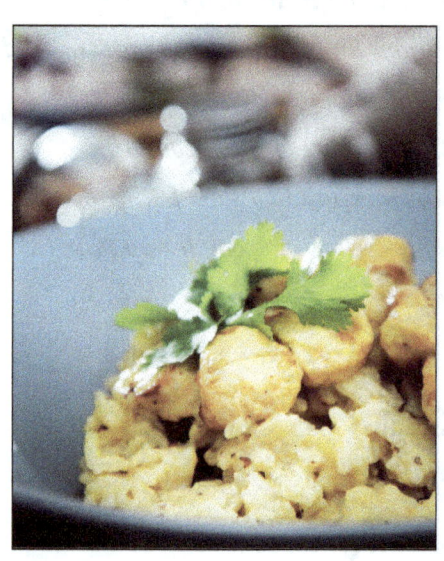

THE DELICIOUS TURKEY WRAP

Preparation time: 10 min
Cooking time: 10 min
Portions: 6
Ingredients:
1 ¼ pounds ground turkey, lean
4 green onions, chopped
1 tbsp olive oil
1 clove of garlic, chopped
2 tsp of chilli paste
8 ounces of water chestnuts, diced
Ingredients:
3 tbsps of hoisin sauce
2 tbsps of coconut amino acids
1 tbsp rice vinegar
12 lettuce leaves with almond butter
1/8 tsp sunflower seeds
Directions:
Take a frying pan and put it over medium heat, add the turkey and garlic to the pan.
Heat for 6 min until cooked through.
Take a bowl and transfer the turkey to it.
Add the onions and water chestnuts.
Mix the hoisin sauce, coconut amino acid, vinegar and chilli paste.
Mix well and transfer to lettuce leaves. Serve and enjoy!

ZOODLES WITH CHICKEN AND BASIL

Preparation time: 10 min
Cooking time: 10 min
Portions: 3
Ingredients:
2 chicken fillets, diced
2 tbsps of ghee
1 pound tomatoes, diced
½ cup basil, chopped
Ingredients:
¼ cup of almond milk
1 clove of garlic, peeled, chopped
1 courgette, chopped
Directions:
Fry the diced chicken in ghee until no longer pink.
Add the tomatoes and season with sunflower seeds.
Bring to the boil and reduce the liquid.
Prepare the Zoodles by chopping the courgettes in a food processor.
Add the basil, garlic, coconut and almond milk to the chicken and cook for a few min.

BAKED CHICKEN WITH PARMESAN

Preparation time: 5 min
Cooking time: 20 min

Portions: *2*

Ingredients:

2 tbsps of ghee

2 boneless chicken breasts, skinless Pink sunflower seeds Freshly ground black pepper

½ cup low-fat mayonnaise

Ingredients:

¼ cup Parmesan cheese, grated

1 tbsp of dry, low-fat, low-sodium Italian seasoning

¼ cup of crushed pork rind

Directions:

Preheat the oven to 425 degrees F. Take a large baking tray and coat with ghee.

Dry the chicken breasts and wrap them with a towel. Season with sunflower seeds and pepper.

Place in the baking tray.

Take a small bowl and add the mayonnaise, Parmesan cheese and Italian dressing.

Spread the mayonnaise mixture evenly over the chicken breast. Sprinkle with the crushed pork rind.

Bake for 20 min until the topping is golden brown. Serve and enjoy!

CRAZY JAPANESE POTATO AND BEEF CROQUETTES

Preparation time: *10 min*
Cooking time: *20 min*

Portions: 10

Ingredients:

3 medium russet potatoes, peeled and cut into pieces

1 tbsp almond butter

1 tbsp vegetable oil

3 onions, diced

Ingredients:

¾ pound of ground beef

4 tsp of light coconut amino acids Multipurpose flour for coating

2 eggs, beaten Panko breadcrumbs for coating

½ cup of frying oil

Directions:

Take a saucepan and place it over medium-high heat; add the potatoes and sunflower seed water and boil for 16 min.

Remove the water and put the potatoes in another bowl, add the almond butter and mash the potatoes.

Take a frying pan and put it over medium heat, add 1 tbsp of oil and let it warm up.

Add the onions and fry until tender. Add the beef coconut amino acid to the onions.

Continue frying until the beef is browned. Mix the beef with the potatoes evenly.

Take another frying pan and put it over medium heat; add half a cup of oil.

Form croquettes with the mashed potato mixture and

cover them with flour, then egg and finally breadcrumbs.

Fry the croquettes until golden brown on all sides. Enjoy your meal!

GOLDEN AUBERGINE CHIPS

Preparation time: *10 min*
Cooking time: *15 min*
Portions: 8
Ingredients:
2 eggs
2 cups of almond flour
Ingredients:
2 tbsps coconut oil, spray
2 aubergines, peeled and thinly sliced Sunflower seeds and pepper
Directions:
Preheat the oven to 400 degrees F.
Take a bowl and mix the sunflower seeds and black pepper.
Take another bowl and beat the eggs until frothy.
Dip the aubergine pieces in the eggs.
Then cover them with the flour mixture.
Add another layer of flour and eggs.
Then, take a baking tray and grease the top with coconut oil.
Cook for about 15 min. Serve and enjoy!

VERY WILD MUSHROOMS PILAF

Preparation time: 10 min
Cooking time: 3 hours
Portions: 4
Ingredients:
1 cup of wild rice
2 cloves of garlic, minced
6 green onions, chopped
Ingredients:
2 tbsps of olive oil
½ pound of baby Bella mushrooms
2 cups of water
Directions:
Add the rice, garlic, onion, oil, mushrooms and water to your Slow Cooker.
Stir well until combined.
Put the lid on and cook on LOW for 3 hours.
Mix the pilaf and divide it between the serving plates. Enjoy your meal!

SPORTS CARROTS FOR CHILDREN

Preparation time: 5 min
Cooking time: 5 min
Portions: 4
Ingredients:

1 lb. baby carrots
1 cup of water
Ingredients:
1 tbsp clarified ghee
1 tbsp chopped fresh mint leaves Flavoured sea vinegar, if required

Directions:

Put a steamer basket on top of your pot and add the carrots. Add the water.

Close the lid and cook at HIGH pressure for 2 min. Make a quick release.

Pass the carrots through a sieve and drain. Clean the insert.

Put the insert back into the cooker and set the cooker to Sauté mode. Add the clarified butter and let it melt.

Add the mint and fry for 30 seconds. Add the carrots to the insert and fry well.

GARDEN SALAD

Preparation time: *5 min*
Cooking time: *20 min*
Portions: 6
Ingredients:
1 pound raw peanuts in shell
1 bay leaf
2 medium-sized tomatoes cut into pieces

½ cup of diced green pepper

½ cup diced sweet onion

Ingredients:

¼ cup diced chilli peppers

¼ cup diced celery

2 tbsps of olive oil

¾ tsp of flavoured vinegar

¼ tsp freshly ground black pepper

Directions:

Boil your peanuts for 1 minute and rinse them.

The skin will be soft, so discard it.

Add 2 cups of water to the Instant Pot. Add the bay leaf and peanuts.

Close the lid and cook at high pressure for 20 min. Drain off the water.

Take a large bowl and add the peanuts and diced vegetables.

Whisk the olive oil, lemon juice and pepper in another bowl.

Pour the mixture over the salad and toss. Enjoy your meal!

OVEN-SMOKED BROCCOLI WITH GARLIC

Preparation time:
Cooking time:
Portions:
Ingredients:

cooking spray

1 tbsp extra virgin olive oil

3 cloves of garlic, minced

1/2 tsp of sea salt

1/4 tsp ground black pepper

Ingredients:

½ tsp of cumin

½ tsp of annatto seeds

3 1/2 cups of sliced broccoli

1 lime, cut into wedges

1 tbsp fresh coriander, chopped

Directions:

Preheat the oven to 450 degrees F. Line a baking tray with aluminium foil and grease with olive oil.

Mix the olive oil, garlic, cumin, annatto seeds, salt and pepper in a bowl.

Add the cauliflower, carrots and broccoli and combine until well coated. Spread them out in a single layer on the baking tray.

Add the lime wedges. Roast in the oven until the vegetables caramelise, about 25 min.

Remove the lime wedges and add the coriander.

ROASTED CAULIFLOWER AND LIMA BEANS

Preparation time:
Cooking time:
Portions:

Ingredients:
cooking spray
1 tbsp vegan butter/melted margarine
9 cloves of garlic, minced
1/2 tsp of sea salt
1/4 tsp ground black pepper
Ingredients:
1 1/2 cups of sliced cauliflower
3 1/2 cups of cherry tomatoes
1 (15-ounce) can lima beans, drained
1 lemon, cut into wedges
Directions:
Preheat the oven to 450 degrees F. Line a baking tray with aluminium foil and grease with melted vegan butter or margarine.
Mix the olive oil, garlic, salt and pepper in a bowl.
Add the cauliflower, tomatoes and lima beans. Spread them in a single layer on the baking tray.
Add the lemon wedges.
Roast in the oven until the vegetables caramelise, about 25 min. Remove the lemon wedges.

Thai Spicy Roasted Black Beans and Choy Sum

Preparation time:
Cooking time:
Portions:
Ingredients:
1 tbsp sesame oil

3 cloves of garlic, minced
1/2 tsp of sea salt
1 tbsp of Thai chilli paste
1/4 tsp ground black pepper

Ingredients:
3 1/2 cups of Choy Sum, coarsely chopped
2 1/2 cups of cherry tomatoes
1 (15-ounce) can black beans, drained
1 lime, cut into wedges
1 tbsp fresh coriander, chopped

Directions:
Preheat the oven to 450 degrees F. Line a baking tray with aluminium foil and grease it with sesame oil.
Mix the olive oil, garlic, salt, Thai chilli paste and pepper in a bowl.
Add the choy sum, tomatoes and black beans.
Spread them out in a single layer on the baking tray.
Add the lime wedges. Roast in the oven until the vegetables caramelise, about 25 min.
Remove the lime wedges and add the coriander.

SIMPLE ROASTED BROCCOLI AND CAULIFLOWER

Preparation time:
Cooking time:
Portions:
Ingredients:

1 tbsp extra virgin olive oil

3 cloves of garlic, minced

1/2 tsp of sea salt

1/4 tsp ground black pepper

Ingredients:

3 1/2 cups of broccoli

2 1/2 cups of cauliflower

1 tbsp chopped fresh thyme

Directions:

Preheat the oven to 450 degrees F.

Line a baking tray with aluminium foil and grease it with olive oil. Mix the olive oil, garlic, salt and pepper in a bowl.

Add the cauliflower and tomatoes and combine until well coated.

Spread them out in a single layer on the baking tray.

Roast in the oven until the vegetables caramelise, about 25 min. Cover with thyme. Simple

ROASTED NAPA CABBAGE AND EXTRA TURNIPS

Preparation time:

Cooking time:

Portions:

Ingredients:

cooking spray

1 tbsp extra virgin olive oil

1/2 tsp of sea salt

Ingredients:
1/4 tsp ground black pepper
1/2 Napa cabbage, medium, thinly sliced
1 medium turnip, thinly sliced

Directions:
Preheat the oven to 450 degrees F.
Line a baking tray with aluminium foil and grease with olive oil.
Mix the extra ingredients well.
Add the main ingredients and combine until well coated.
Spread in a single layer on the baking tray.
Roast in the oven until the vegetables caramelise, about 25 min.

Simple roasted cabbage with artichoke heart and extra choy sum

Preparation time:
Cooking time:
Portions:

Ingredients:
1 tbsp extra virgin olive oil
1/2 tsp of sea salt
1/4 tsp ground black pepper Main ingredients

Ingredients:
1 bunch of cabbage, rinsed and drained
1 cup of canned artichoke hearts
1/2 medium-flowered Chinese cabbage (choy sum), roughly chopped

Directions:
Preheat the oven to 450 degrees F. Line a baking tray with aluminium foil and grease with olive oil.
Mix the extra ingredients well.
Add the main ingredients and combine until well coated.
Spread in a single layer on the baking tray.
Roast in the oven until the vegetables caramelise, about 25 min.

ROASTED CABBAGE AND BOK CHOY EXTRA

Preparation time:
Cooking time:
Portions:
Ingredients:
1 tbsp extra virgin olive oil
1/2 tsp of sea salt
1/4 tsp ground black pepper
Ingredients:
1 bunch of cabbage, rinsed and drained
1 bunch of bok choy, rinsed, drained and coarsely chopped
Directions:
Preheat the oven to 450 degrees F.
Line a baking tray with aluminium foil and grease with olive oil.
Mix the extra ingredients well.

Add the main ingredients and combine until well coated.
Spread in a single layer on the baking tray.
Roast in the oven until the vegetables caramelise, about 25 min.

ROASTED SOYA BEANS AND WINTER SQUASH

Preparation time:
Cooking time:
Portions:
Ingredients:
2 (15-ounce) cans of soya, rinsed and drained
1/2 winter squash - peeled, seeded and cut into 1 inch pieces 1 red onion, diced
1 sweet potato, peeled and cut into 1-inch cubes
2 large carrots, cut into 1 inch pieces
3 medium-sized potatoes
4 tbsps extra virgin olive oil Ingredients for the dressing
Ingredients:
1 tsp salt
1/2 tsp ground black pepper
1 tsp of onion powder
1 tsp dried basil
1 tsp of Italian seasoning Ingredients for the toppings
2 green onions, chopped (optional)
Directions:

Preheat the oven to 350 degrees F.

Grease the baking tray. Combine the beans, pumpkin, onion, sweet potato, carrots and russet potatoes on the prepared baking tray. Drizzle with oil and stir to coat.

Combine the dressing ingredients in a bowl, spread over the vegetables on the baking tray and stir to coat them with the dressing.

Bake for 25 min. Stir often until the vegetables are soft and lightly browned and the beans are crispy, about 20-25 min more.

Season with more salt and black pepper to taste, add green onion before serving.

ROASTED MUSHROOMS AND PUMPKIN

Preparation time*:*
Cooking time:
Portions:
Ingredients:
2 (15-ounce) cans of button mushrooms, rinsed and drained
1/2 summer squash - peeled, seeded and cut into 1-inch pieces
1 red onion, diced
2 large turnips, cut into 1-inch pieces
2 large parsnips, cut into 1 inch pieces
3 medium-sized potatoes, cut into 1-inch pieces

3 tbsps butter Ingredients for the dressing

Ingredients:

1 tsp salt

1/2 tsp ground black pepper

1 tsp of onion powder

2 tsp of garlic powder

1 tsp of Herbes de Provence Ingredients for the toppings

2 sprigs of thyme, chopped (optional)

Directions:

Preheat the oven to 350 degrees F.

Grease the baking tray. Combine the main ingredients on the prepared baking tray.

Drizzle with melted butter or margarine and stir to coat. Combine the ingredients for the dressing in a bowl, spread over the vegetables on the baking tray and stir to coat them with the dressing.

Cook for 25 min. Stir frequently until the vegetables are soft and lightly browned and the chickpeas are crispy, about another 20-25 min.

Season with more salt and black pepper to taste, add thyme before serving.

RUTABAGA ROASTED TOMATOES AND KOHLRABI

Preparation time:
Cooking time:
Portions:

Ingredients:

3 large tomatoes, cut into 1 inch pieces

3 red onion, diced

1 rutabaga, peeled and cut into 1-inch cubes

2 large carrots, cut into 1 inch pieces

3 medium-sized kohlrabi, cut into 1-inch pieces

3 tbsps extra virgin olive oil Ingredients for the dressing

1 tsp salt

Ingredients:

1/2 tsp ground black pepper

1 tsp onion powder

2 tsp of garlic powder

1 tsp Spanish paprika

1 tsp of cumin Ingredients for the toppings

2 sprigs of parsley, chopped (optional)

Directions:

Preheat oven to 350 degrees F. Grease baking tray. Combine main ingredients on prepared baking sheet.

Drizzle with oil and stir to coat. Combine the dressing ingredients in a bowl, spread over the vegetables on the baking tray and stir to coat them with the dressing.

Bake for 25 min. Stir often until the vegetables are soft, about 20-25 min more.

Season with more salt and black pepper to taste, add parsley before serving.

ROASTED BRUSSELS SPROUTS AND BROCCOLI

Preparation time:
Cooking time:
Portions:
Ingredients:
1 large broccoli, sliced
1 cup of bean sprouts
1 red onion, diced
3 large kohlrabi, cut into 1 inch pieces
2 large carrots, cut into 1 inch pieces
3 medium-sized potatoes, cut into 1-inch pieces
3 tbsps extra virgin olive oil Ingredients for the dressing
Ingredients:
1 tsp salt
1/2 tsp ground black pepper
1 tsp of onion powder
2 tsp of garlic powder
1 tsp of ground fennel seeds
1 tsp dry rubbed sage Ingredients for the toppings
2 green onions, chopped (optional)
Directions:
Preheat the oven to 350 degrees F. Grease the baking tray.
Combine the main ingredients on the prepared baking tray. Drizzle with oil and stir to coat.
Combine the dressing ingredients in a bowl, spread

over the vegetables on the baking tray and stir to coat them with the dressing. Bake in the oven for 25 min.

Stir frequently until the vegetables are soft and lightly browned and the chickpeas are crispy, about 20-25 min more.

Season with more salt and black pepper to taste, add green onion before serving.

ROASTED BROCCOLI, SWEET POTATOES AND BEAN SPROUTS

Preparation time:
Cooking time:
Portions:
Ingredients:
1 large broccoli, sliced
1 cup of bean sprouts
1 yellow onion, diced
1 sweet potato, peeled and cut into 1-inch cubes
2 large carrots, cut into 1 inch pieces
3 medium-sized potatoes, cut into 1-inch pieces
3 tbsps canola oil Ingredients for the dressing
Ingredients:
1 tsp salt
1/2 tsp ground black pepper
1 tsp of onion powder
2 tsp of garlic powder
½ cup of grated gouda cheese

¼ cup Parmesan cheese

2 green onions, chopped (optional)

Directions:

Preheat oven to 350 degrees F. Grease baking dish. Combine main ingredients on prepared baking sheet. Drizzle with oil and toss to coat.

Combine the dressing ingredients in a bowl, spread over the vegetables on the baking tray and stir to coat them with the dressing. Bake in the oven for 25 min.

Stir often until the vegetables are soft and lightly browned and the chickpeas are crispy, about another 20-25 min.

Season with more salt and black pepper to taste, add green onion before serving.

SWEET POTATOES AND ROASTED RED BEETS

Preparation time:

Cooking time:

Portions:

Ingredients:

1 ½ cups of Brussels sprouts, chopped

1 cup large sweet potatoes, chopped

1 cup large carrots, chopped

1 ½ cups of broccoli florets

Ingredients:

1 cup diced red beets

1/2 cup yellow onion, chopped
2 tbsps sesame seed oil salt and ground black pepper to taste

Directions:
Preheat the oven to 425 degrees F (220 degrees C).
Set the rack to the second lowest level of the oven. Pour lightly salted water into a bowl.
Soak the Brussels sprouts in salted water for 15 min and drain.
Place the rest of the ingredients in a bowl.
Spread the vegetables in a single layer on a baking tray.
Roast in the oven until the vegetables begin to brown and cook, about 45 min.

BEETROOT AND BROCCOLI FLORETS BAKED SICHUAN STYLE

Preparation time:
Cooking time:
Portions:
Ingredients:
1 ½ cups Brussels sprouts, chopped
1 cup of broccoli florets
1 cup Choggia beets, chopped
1½ cups of cauliflower florets
Ingredients:
1 cup mushrooms, sliced
1/2 cup chopped red onion

2 tbsps of sesame oil

½ tsp Sichuan pepper salt Ground black pepper to taste

Directions:

Preheat the oven to 425 degrees F (220 degrees C).

Set the rack to the second lowest level of the oven. Pour lightly salted water into a bowl.

Soak the Brussels sprouts in salted water for 15 min and drain. Put the rest of the ingredients in a bowl.

Spread the vegetables in a single layer on a baking tray.

BAKED ENOKI AND MINI CABBAGE

Preparation time:
Cooking time:
Portions:
Ingredients:
1 ½ cups mini cabbage, chopped
1 cup of broccoli florets
1 cup enoki mushrooms, sliced
1½ cups of cauliflower florets
Ingredients:
1 cup oyster mushrooms
1/2 cup chopped red onion
2 tbsps olive oil salt and ground black pepper to taste
Directions:

Preheat the oven to 425 degrees F (220 degrees C).
Set the rack to the second lowest level of the oven.
Pour lightly salted water into a bowl. Soak the Brussels sprouts in salted water for 15 min and drain.
Place the rest of the ingredients in a bowl.
Spread the vegetables in a single layer on a baking tray.
Roast in the oven until the vegetables begin to brown and cook, about 45 min.

TRIPLE ROASTED MUSHROOMS

Preparation time:
Cooking time:
Portions:
Ingredients:
2 cups spinach, rinsed
1 cup oyster mushrooms
1 cup mushrooms, sliced
1 ½ cups of enoki mushrooms
Ingredients:
1/2 cup chopped red onion
2 tbsps extra virgin olive oil salt and ground black pepper to taste
1/4 cup cottage cheese
Directions:
Preheat the oven to 425 degrees F (220 degrees C).

Set the rack to the second lowest level of the oven.
Pour lightly salted water into a bowl.
Soak the spinach in salted water for 15 min and drain.
Place the rest of the ingredients in a bowl.
Spread the vegetables in a single layer on a baking tray. Roast in the oven until the vegetables begin to brown and cook, about 45 min.

MINI ROAST CABBAGE AND SWEET POTATOES

Preparation time:
Cooking time:
Portions:
Ingredients:
1 ½ cups mini cabbage, cut up
1 cup of large pieces of potatoes
1 cup of large pieces of rainbow carrots
1 ½ cups of potato pieces
Ingredients:
1 cup parsnips
1/2 cup of red onion pieces
2 tbsps extra virgin olive oil Sea salt Rainbow pepper to taste
1/4 cup cottage cheese
Directions:
Preheat the oven to 425 degrees F (220 degrees C).
Set the rack to the second lowest level of the oven.
Pour lightly salted water into a bowl.

Soak the mini cabbages in salted water for 15 min and drain.

Put the rest of the ingredients in a bowl. Spread the vegetables in a single layer on a baking tray.

Roast in the oven until the vegetables begin to brown and cook, about 45 min.

ROASTED RED POTATOES AND ASPARAGUS

Preparation time*:*
Cooking time:
Portions:
Ingredients:
1 1/2 pounds red potatoes, cut into pieces
2 tbsps of extra virgin olive oil
12 garlic cloves, thinly sliced
1 tbsp and 1 tsp of dried rosemary
Ingredients:
4 tsp dried thyme
2 tsp of sea salt
1 bunch of fresh asparagus, trimmed and cut into 1-inch pieces
Directions:
Preheat the oven to 425 degrees F.

In a baking dish, combine the first 5 ingredients and 1/2 of the sea salt. Cover with aluminium foil.

Cook for 20 min in the oven. Add the asparagus, oil

and salt. Cover and cook for about 15 min, or until the potatoes are tender.

Increase the oven temperature to 450 degrees F.

Remove the aluminium foil and bake for 8 min, until the potatoes are lightly browned.

Green beans roasted in butter with garlic and lime

Preparation time:

Cooking time:

Portions:

Ingredients:

1 1/2 lb potatoes, cut into pieces

4 tbsps of butter

12 garlic cloves, thinly sliced

Ingredients:

2 tbsps of lime juice

2 tsp of sea salt

1 bunch of fresh green beans, trimmed and cut into 1-inch pieces

Directions:

Preheat the oven to 425 degrees F. In a baking dish, combine the first 5 ingredients and 1/2 of the sea salt.

Cover with aluminium foil. Cook for 20 min in the oven. Add the green beans, oil and salt.

Cover and bake for about 15 min, or until the potatoes become tender. Increase the oven temperature to 450 degrees F.

Remove the aluminium foil and bake for 8 min, until the potatoes are lightly browned.

ROASTED ESCAROLE AND HEARTS OF PALM

Preparation time:
Cooking time:
Portions:
Ingredients:
1 1/2 pounds escarole, cut into chunks
3 tbsps of extra virgin olive oil
12 garlic cloves, thinly sliced
Ingredients:
1 tbsp and 1 tsp of dried rosemary
4 tsp dried thyme
2 tsp of sea salt
1 bunch of hearts of palm, trimmed and cut into 1 inch pieces
Directions:
Preheat the oven to 425 degrees F. In a baking dish, combine the first 5 ingredients and 1/2 of the sea salt.
Cover with aluminium foil. Cook for 20 min in the oven. Add the hearts of palm, oil and salt.
Cover and bake for about 15 min, or until escarole is tender. Increase the oven temperature to 450 degrees F.

Remove the aluminium foil and bake for 8 min, until the potatoes are lightly browned.

ROASTED ITALIAN CABBAGE AND ASPARAGUS

Preparation time:
Cooking time:
Portions:
Ingredients:
1 1/2 pounds kohlrabi, chopped
2 tbsps of extra virgin olive oil
12 garlic cloves, thinly sliced
1 tbsp of Italian seasoning
Ingredients:
4 tsp dried thyme
2 tsp of sea salt
1 bunch of fresh asparagus, trimmed and cut into 1-inch pieces
Directions:
Preheat the oven to 425 degrees F. In a baking dish, combine the first 5 ingredients and 1/2 of the sea salt.
Cover with aluminium foil. Bake for 20 min in the oven.
Add the asparagus, oil and salt.
Cover and bake for about 15 min, or until the kohlrabi becomes tender. Increase the oven temperature to 450 degrees F.

Remove the foil and bake for 8 min, until the kohlrabi is lightly browned.

ROAST POTATOES AND SWEET POTATOES WITH NUTS

Preparation time*:*
Cooking time:
Portions:
Ingredients:
1/2 pound red potatoes, cut into chunks
½ pound sweet potatoes, cut into chunks
2 tbsps of peanut oil
12 garlic cloves, thinly sliced
Ingredients:
1 tbsp and 1 tsp Herbes de Provence
2 tsp of sea salt
1 bunch of fresh asparagus, trimmed and cut into 1-inch pieces
Directions:
Preheat the oven to 425 degrees F. In a baking dish, combine the first 6 ingredients and 1/2 of the sea salt.
Cover with aluminium foil. Cook for 20 min in the oven. Add the asparagus, oil and salt.
Cover and bake for about 15 min, or until the root vegetables become tender. Increase the oven temperature to 450 degrees F.

Remove the aluminium foil and bake for 8 min, until the potatoes are lightly browned.

BAKED KOHLRABI, YUCCA ROOT AND MUSTARD

Preparation time:
Cooking time:
Portions:
Ingredients:
1/2 pound kohlrabi, chopped
½ pound of yucca root, chopped
½ pound of mustard
2 tbsps of extra virgin olive oil
12 garlic cloves, thinly sliced
Ingredients:
1 tbsp and 1 tsp of dried rosemary
4 tsp dried thyme
2 tsp of sea salt
1 bunch of fresh green beans, trimmed and cut into 1-inch pieces
Directions:
Preheat the oven to 425 degrees F. In a baking dish, combine the first 7 ingredients and 1/2 of the sea salt.
Cover with aluminium foil. Cook for 20 min in the oven. Add the green beans, olive oil and salt.
Cover and bake for about 15 min, or until the root

vegetables become tender. Increase the oven temperature to 450 degrees F.

Remove the aluminium foil and bake for 8 min, until the potatoes are lightly browned.

BAKED PURPLE CABBAGE WITH RAINBOW PEPPERCORNS

Preparation time:
Cooking time:
Portions:
Ingredients:
1 16 oz package of fresh purple cabbage
2 small red onions, thinly sliced
1/2 cup and 1 tbsp extra virgin olive oil, divided
1/4 tsp sea salt
Ingredients:
1/4 tsp of rainbow pepper
1 shallot, chopped
1/4 cup balsamic vinegar
1 tsp Herbes de Provence
Directions:
Preheat the oven to 425 degrees F (220 degrees C).

Grease a baking tray. Combine the cabbage and onion in a bowl.

Add 4 tbsps of olive oil, the salt and the peppercorns Mix to coat and spread the sprout mixture on the baking tray.

Cook until the sprouts and onion are tender, about

25-30 min. Heat the remaining tbsp of olive oil in a small frying pan over medium-high heat. Fry the shallots until tender, about 5 min.

Add the balsamic vinegar and cook until the glaze is reduced, about 5 min.

Add the Herbes de Provence to the balsamic glaze and pour over the sprouts.

BAKED CRIMINI MUSHROOMS AND RED POTATOES

***Preparation time**:*
Cooking time:
Portions:
Ingredients:
1 pound red potatoes, cut in half
2 tbsps of extra virgin olive oil
1/2 pound cremini mushrooms
8 cloves of garlic, unpeeled
2 tbsps chopped fresh thyme
Ingredients:
1 tbsp extra virgin olive oil sea salt and ground black pepper to taste
1/4 pound of cherry tomatoes
3 tbsps of toasted pine nuts
1/4 pound spinach, thinly sliced
Directions:
Preheat the oven to 425 degrees F. Spread the potatoes

in a pan with 2 tbsps of olive oil and roast for 15 min, turning once.

Add the mushrooms, stem side up Add the garlic cloves to the pan and cook until lightly golden Sprinkle with thyme

Drizzle with 1 tbsp of olive oil and season with sea salt and black pepper.

Return to the oven and bake for 5 min. Add the cherry tomatoes to the pan. Return to the oven and bake until the mushrooms are softened, 5 min.

Sprinkle the pine nuts over the potatoes and mushrooms. Serve with spinach.

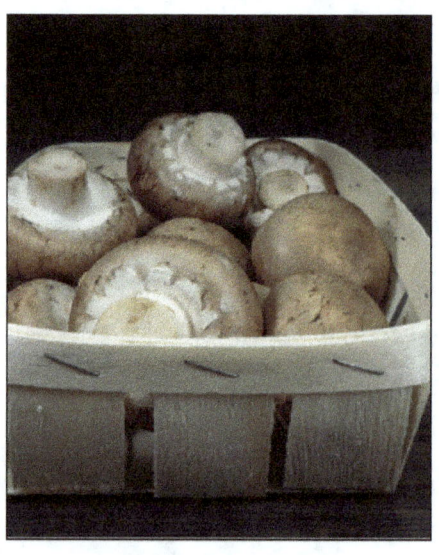

CHAMPIGNON MUSHROOMS AND BAKED SUMMER SQUASH

Preparation time:

Cooking time:
Portions:

Ingredients:

1 pound summer squash, halved

2 tbsps of extra virgin olive oil

1/2 pound mushrooms

8 cloves of garlic, unpeeled

2 tbsps of cumin

1 tbsp annatto seeds

Ingredients:

½ tbsp cayenne pepper

1 tbsp extra virgin olive oil sea salt and ground black pepper to taste

1/4 pound of cherry tomatoes

3 tbsps of toasted pine nuts

1/4 pound spinach, thinly sliced

Directions:

Preheat the oven to 425 degrees F. Spread the summer squash in a pan with 2 tbsps of olive oil and roast for 15 min, turning once.

Add the mushrooms with the stem upwards Add the garlic cloves to the pan and cook until lightly golden Sprinkle with cumin, cayenne pepper and annatto seeds.

Drizzle with 1 tbsp of olive oil and season with sea salt and black pepper.

Return to the oven and bake for 5 min. Add the cherry tomatoes to the pan.

Return to the oven and bake until the mushrooms have softened, 5 min.

Sprinkle the summer squash and mushrooms with pine nuts. Serve with spinach.

ROASTED WATERCRESS AND SUMMER SQUASH

Preparation time:
Cooking time:
Portions:
Ingredients:
1 1/2 pounds of summer squash, peeled and cut into 1-inch pieces
½ red onion, thinly sliced
¼ cup of water
½ vegetable stock cube, crumbled
1 tbsp sesame oil
Ingredients:
½ tsp of 5 Chinese spice powder
½ tsp of Sichuan pepper
½ tsp of chilli powder Black pepper
½ pound fresh watercress, coarsely chopped
Directions:
Put all the ingredients in a saucepan over low heat, except the last one.
Add a handful of watercress and fill the pot over a low heat. If you can't put everything in at once,

let the first batch cook first and add more watercress.

Cook for 3 to 4 hours on a medium heat until the summer squash is soft. Scrape down the sides and serve.

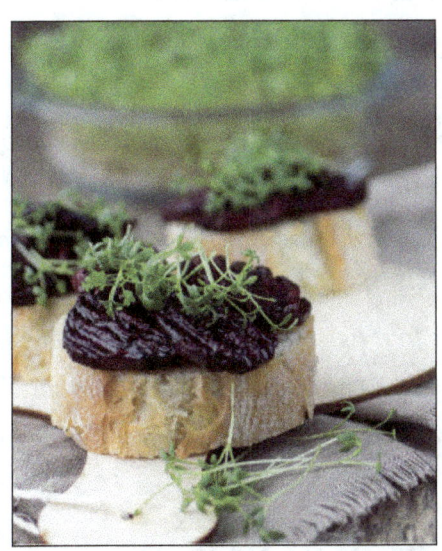

BUTTERED POTATOES AND SPINACH

Preparation time:
Cooking time:
Portions:
Ingredients:
1 1/2 pounds of red potatoes, peeled and cut into 1-inch pieces
½ onion, thinly sliced
¼ cup of water

½ vegetable stock cube, crumbled

2 tbsps of salted butter

Ingredients:

½ tsp Herbes de Provence

½ tsp of thyme

½ tsp of chilli powder Black pepper

½ pound fresh spinach, coarsely chopped

Directions:

Put all the ingredients in a saucepan over low heat, except the last one.

Top with handfuls of spinach and fill the pot over a low heat. If you cannot put everything in at once, let the first batch cook first and add more spinach.

Cook for 3 to 4 hours on a medium heat until the potatoes are soft. Scrape down the sides and serve.

SMOKED ROASTED BEETROOT AND CAULIFLOWER

Preparation time:
Cooking time:
Portions:

Ingredients:

1 1/2 lbs. cauliflower, peeled and cut into 1 inch pieces

½ red onion, thinly sliced

¼ cup of water

½ vegetable stock cube, crumbled

1 tbsp extra virgin olive oil

Ingredients:

½ tsp of cumin

½ tsp of chilli powder Black pepper

½ pound of fresh beets, coarsely chopped

Directions:

Put all the ingredients in a saucepan over low heat, except the last one.

Add a handful of Swiss chard and fill the pot over a low heat. If you can't put everything in at once, let the first batch cook first and add more chard.

Cook for 3 to 4 hours on a medium heat until the potatoes are soft.

Scrape down the sides and serve.

ROASTED SPINACH AND BROCCOLI WITH JALAPENO

Preparation time:
Cooking time:
Portions:

Ingredients:

1 1/2 lb. broccoli florets

½ onion, thinly sliced

¼ cup of water

½ vegetable stock cube, crumbled

1 tbsp extra virgin olive oil

Ingredients:

½ tsp of cumin

8 jalapeno peppers, finely chopped

1 ancho chilli

½ tsp of chilli powder black pepper
½ pound fresh spinach, coarsely chopped
Directions:
Put all the ingredients in a saucepan over low heat, except the last one.
Top with handfuls of spinach and fill the pot over a low heat. If you cannot put everything in at once, let the first batch cook first and add more spinach.
Cook for 3 to 4 hours on a medium heat until the broccoli is tender.
Scrape down the sides and serve.

OMELETTE WITH ONIONS AND MUSHROOMS

Preparation time: 15 min
Cooking time:
Portions: 2
Ingredients:
4 eggs, beaten
1 cup mushrooms, sliced
2 tbsps of olive oil, divided by
Ingredients:
1 clove of garlic, minced Salt and black pepper to taste
¼ cup of sliced onions
Directions:
Heat the olive oil in a frying pan over medium heat.
Add the garlic, mushrooms and onions.

Cook for 6 min, stirring frequently. Season with salt and pepper. Increase the heat and cook for 3 min.
Remove to a plate. In the same pan, add the eggs and make sure they are evenly distributed.
Add the vegetables. Cut into slices and serve.

GREEN CITRUS JUICE

Preparation time: 5 min
Cooking time:
Portions: 1
Ingredients:
½ grapefruit
½ lemon
3 cups of cabbage
1 cucumber
Ingredients:
¼ cup of fresh parsley leaves
¼ cup of pineapple, cut into wedges
½ green apple
1 tsp freshly grated ginger
Directions:
In a blender, place the cabbage, parsley, cucumber, pineapple, grapefruit, apple, lemon and ginger and blend until smooth.
Serve in a tall glass.

COURGETTE AND EGG NESTS WITH CHILLIES

Preparation time: 25 min
Cooking time:
Portions: 4
Ingredients:
4 eggs
2 tbsps of olive oil
1 lb. courgettes, shredded Salt and black pepper to taste
Ingredients:
½ red pepper, seeded and chopped
2 tbsps chopped parsley
Directions:
Preheat the oven to 360 F. Combine the courgettes, salt, pepper and olive oil in a bowl.
Form nests with a spoon on a greased baking tray.
Break an egg into each nest and season with salt, pepper and chilli. Cook for 11 min.
Serve topped with parsley.

OATS WITH CHIA AND BANANA

Preparation time: 10 min
Cooking time:
Portions:
Ingredients:
½ cup walnuts, chopped

1 banana, peeled and sliced
1 cup of Greek yoghurt
Ingredients:
2 dates, pitted and chopped
1 cup rolled oats
2 tbsps of chia seeds
Directions:
Place the banana, yoghurt, dates, cocoa powder, oats and chia seeds in a bowl and blend until smooth.

Leave to rest for 1 hour and spoon onto a bowl. Sprinkle with walnuts and serve.

PARMESAN OMELETTE

Preparation time: 5 min
Cooking time: 10 min
Portions: 2
Ingredients:
1 tbsp cream cheese
2 eggs, beaten
¼ tsp of paprika
½ tsp dried oregano
Ingredients:
¼ tsp of dried dill
1 oz Parmesan cheese, grated
1 tsp of coconut oil
Directions:

Mix the cream cheese with the eggs, dried oregano and dill.
Put the coconut oil in a frying pan and heat it until it covers the whole pan.
Then pour the egg mixture into the pan and flatten it.
Add the grated Parmesan cheese and close the lid.
Cook the omelette for 10 min over a low heat.
Then transfer the cooked omelette to a serving dish and sprinkle with paprika.

WATERMELON PIZZA

Preparation time: 10 min
Cooking time:
Portions: 2
Ingredients:
9 ounces of watermelon slice
1 tbsp pomegranate sauce

Ingredients:
2 ounces of feta cheese, crumbled
1 tbsp fresh coriander, chopped

Directions:
Place the watermelon slice on the plate and sprinkle with the crumbled feta cheese.
Add the fresh coriander. After this, sprinkle the pizza generously with pomegranate juice.

Cut the pizza into portions.

AVOCADO MILKSHAKE

Preparation time: 10 min
Cooking time:
Portions: 3
Ingredients:
1 avocado, peeled and stoned
2 tbsps of liquid honey
½ tsp of vanilla extract
Ingredients:
½ cup double cream
1 cup of milk
1/3 cup ice cubes
Directions:
Chop the avocado and put it in the food processor.
Add the liquid honey, vanilla extract, double cream, milk and ice cubes. Blend the mixture until smooth.
Pour the cooked smoothie into serving glasses.

CAULIFLOWER FRITTERS

Preparation time: 10 min
Cooking time: 10 min
Portions: 2

Ingredients:
1 cup cauliflower, shredded
1 egg, beaten
1 tbsp whole wheat flour
Ingredients:
1 oz grated Parmesan cheese
½ tsp ground black pepper
1 tbsp canola oil
Directions:
In a bowl, mix together the shredded cauliflower and the egg. Add the wheat flour, grated Parmesan cheese and ground black pepper.
Stir the mixture with the help of a fork until smooth and homogeneous.
Pour the canola oil into the pan and bring it to the boil. Cut out pancakes from the cauliflower mixture with the help of your fingertips or a spoon and transfer them to the hot oil.
Roast the pancakes for 4 min on each side over medium-low heat.

COCOA OATMEAL

Preparation time: 10 min
Cooking time: 15 min
Portions: 2
Ingredients:
1 ½ cups oatmeal

1 tbsp of cocoa powder

½ cup double cream

¼ cup of water

Ingredients:

1 tsp of vanilla extract

1 tbsp butter

2 tbsps of Splenda

Directions:

Mix the oatmeal with the cocoa powder and Splenda.

Transfer the mixture to the saucepan, add the vanilla extract, water and double cream.

Stir gently with the help of the spatula. Close the lid and cook for 10-15 min over a medium-low heat.

Remove the cocoa oatmeal from the heat and add the butter. Stir well.

SPANAKOPITA BREAKFAST

Preparation time: 15 min
Cooking time: 1 hour
Portions: 6
Ingredients:
2 cups of spinach
1 white onion, diced
½ cup fresh parsley
1 tsp chopped garlic
3 ounces of feta cheese, crumbled
Ingredients:

1 tsp of paprika powder

2 eggs, beaten

1/3 cup melted butter

2 ounces of phyllo dough

Directions:

Separate the Phyllo dough into 2 parts.

Brush the casserole dish well with butter and place 1 part of the Phyllo dough inside.

Also brush its surface with butter. Put the spinach and fresh parsley in the blender.

Blend until smooth and transfer to the bowl. Add the minced garlic, feta cheese, ground paprika, eggs and diced onion.

Stir well. Pour the spinach mixture into the casserole dish and flatten it well.

Cover the spinach mixture with the remaining Phyllo dough and pour the remaining butter over it.

Bake the spanakopita for 1 hour at 350F. Cut into portions.

FRITATTA OF POBLANO

Preparation time: *10 min*
Cooking time: *15 min*
Portions: 4
Ingredients:
5 eggs, beaten
1 poblano pepper, chopped, raw

1 oz shallot, chopped
1/3 cup double cream
Ingredients:
½ tsp of butter
½ tsp of salt
½ tsp of chilli flakes
1 tbsp fresh coriander, chopped
Directions:
Mix the eggs with the double cream and beat until smooth.
Add chopped chile poblano, shallots, salt, chilli flakes and fresh cilantro.
Put the butter in a frying pan and melt it. Add the egg mixture and flatten it in the pan if necessary.
Close the lid and cook the omelette for 15 min over a medium-low heat. When the omelette is cooked, it will be firm.

QUICK AND EASY STEAK

Preparation time: *15 min*
Cooking time: *10 min*
Portions: 2
Ingredients:
½ pound steak, quality cut
Ingredients:
Salt and freshly cracked black pepper
Directions:

Switch on the air fryer, place the basket for frying, then set the temperature to 385°F and let it preheat.

In the meantime, prepare the steaks, and season them with salt and freshly cracked black pepper on both sides.

When the fryer is preheated, add the prepared steaks to the basket of the fryer, close it with the lid and cook for 15 min.

When finished, transfer the steaks to a plate and serve immediately. To prepare the meal, divide the steaks evenly between two heat-resistant containers, close them with the lid and refrigerate for up to 3 days until ready to serve.

When you are ready to eat, heat the steaks in the microwave until hot and then serve.

Courgette noodles with four cheeses and basil pesto

Preparation time: 10 min
Cooking time: 15 min
Portions: 2
Ingredients:
4 cups of courgette noodles
4 ounces of mascarpone
1/8 cup Romano cheese
2 tbsps grated Parmesan cheese
¼ tsp of salt
Ingredients:

½ tsp ground black pepper

2 1/8 tsp nutmeg powder

1/8 cup basil pesto

½ cup of shredded mozzarella

1 tbsp olive oil

Directions:

Turn on the oven, then set the temperature to 400 °F and let it preheat.

Meanwhile, place the courgette noodles in a heatproof bowl and microwave on high heat for 3 min, set aside until needed. Take another heat-resistant bowl, add all the cheeses except the mozzarella, season with salt, black pepper and nutmeg, and microwave on high heat for 1 minute until the cheese has melted.

Blend the cheese mixture, add the cooked courgette noodles together with the basil pesto and mozzarella and fold until well mixed.

Take a casserole dish, grease it with oil, add the courgette noodle mixture and then bake for 10 min. Serve immediately.

BLUEBERRY AND VANILLA SCONES

Preparation time: 10 min
Cooking time: 10 min
Portions: 12
Ingredients:

1½ cups almond flour

3 organic eggs, beaten

2 tbsps baking powder

½ cup of stevia

Ingredients:

2 tbsps vanilla extract, unsweetened

¾ cup of fresh raspberries

1 tbsp olive oil

Directions:

Turn on the oven, then set the temperature to 375°F and let it preheat.

Take a large bowl, add the flour and eggs, stir in the baking powder, stevia and vanilla until combined and then add the berries.

Take a baking tray, grease it with oil, pour over the batter prepared with an ice cream scoop and bake for 10 min until cooked through.

When finished, transfer the scones to a wire rack, leave to cool completely and then serve.

Chapter Four

DINNER

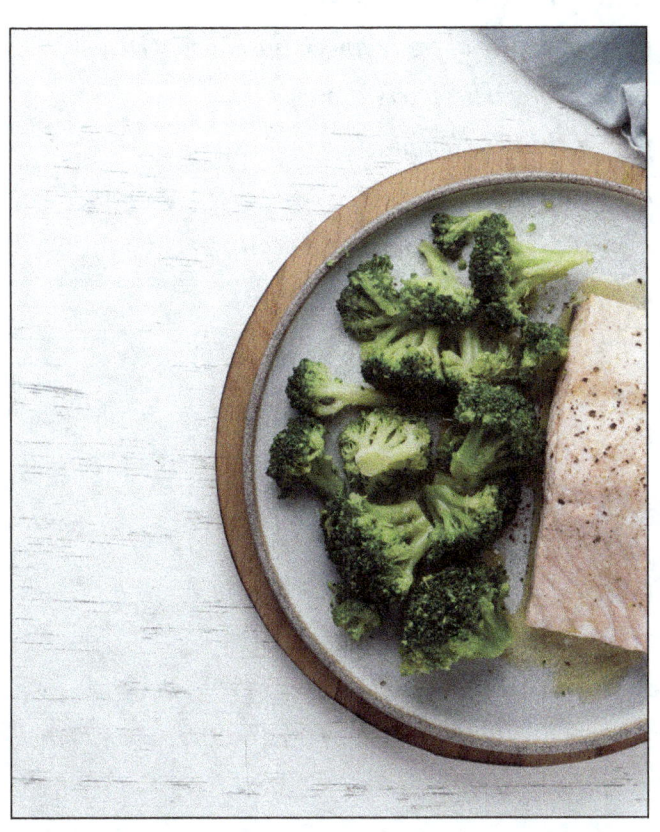

CURRIED BEEF MEATBALLS

***Preparation time**: 20 min*
***Cooking time:** 22 min*
***Portions:** 6*
Ingredients:
For the meatballs:
1 pound lean ground beef
2 organic eggs, bea10
3 tbsps red onion, chopped
¼ cup fresh basil leaves, chopped
1 (1 inch) piece of fresh ginger, finely chopped
4 cloves of garlic, finely chopped
3 Thai chillies, chopped
1 tbsp of coconut sugar
1 tbsp red curry paste - Salt, to taste -
1 tbsp fish sauce
Ingredients:
2 tbsps of coconut oil
For Curry:
1 red onion, chopped - Salt, to taste
4 cloves of garlic, minced
1 piece of fresh ginger (1 inch), chopped
2 Thai chillies, chopped
2 tbsps of red curry paste
1 coconut milk (14 oz) - Salt and freshly ground black pepper, to taste

Lime wedge, for serving

Directions:

For the meatballs in a large bowl, add all the ingredients except the oil and mix until well combined. Make small balls from the mixture. In a large frying pan, melt the coconut oil over medium heat. Add the patties and cook for about 3-5 min or until golden brown on all sides.

Transfer the meatballs to a bowl. In the same pan, add the onion and a pinch of salt and fry for about 5 min. Add the garlic, ginger and chillies and fry for about 1 minute. Add the curry paste and stir-fry for about 1 minute.

Add the coconut milk and meatballs and bring to the boil over low heat. Reduce the heat to low and simmer, covered, for about 10 min. Serve with the lime wedge dressing.

GRILLED STEAK WITH COCONUT

Preparation time: 15 min
Cooking time: 8-9 min
Portions: 4

Ingredients:

2 tsp fresh ginger, finely grated
2 tsp fresh lime zest, finely grated
¼ cup of coconut sugar
2 tsp of fish sauce

Ingredients:

2 tbsps fresh lime juice

½ cup of coconut milk

1 pound of beef skirt steak, trimmed and cut into 4-inch slices lengthwise

Salt, to taste

Directions:

In a resealable bag, mix all the ingredients except the steak and salt. Add the steak and coat generously with the marinade. Seal the bag and refrigerate to marinate for about 4-12 hours. Preheat the grill to high heat. Grease the grill grate. Remove the steak from the fridge and discard the marinade.

Using a paper towel, pat the steak dry and sprinkle it evenly with salt. Cook the steak for about 3 1/2 min. Flip the middle and cook for about 2 1/2 to 5 min or until desired doneness.

Remove from the grill pan and hold the side for about 5 min before slicing. Using a clear, crispy knife, cut into desired slices and serve.

LAMB WITH PRUNES

Preparation time: *15 min*
Cooking time: *a couple of hours and 40 min*
Portions: *4-6*
Ingredients:
3 tbsps of coconut oil

2 onions, finely chopped

1 (1 inch) piece of fresh ginger, chopped

3 cloves of garlic, minced

½ tsp turmeric powder

2 ½ pounds of lamb shoulder, trimmed and cut into 3-inch cubes

Ingredients:

Salt and freshly ground black pepper, to taste

½ tsp of saffron threads, crumbled

1 cinnamon stick

3 cups of water

1 cup runes, pitted and halved

Directions:

In a large frying pan, melt the coconut oil over medium heat. Add the onions, ginger, garlic cloves and turmeric and fry for about 3-5 min. Sprinkle the lamb evenly with salt and black pepper. In the frying pan, add the lamb and saffron threads and cook for about 4-5 min.

Add the cinnamon stick and water and bring to the boil over high heat. Reduce the heat to low and simmer, covered, for about 1½ to 120 min or until the lamb has reached the desired temperature.

Add the plums and simmer for about 20 ½ hours. Remove the cinnamon stick and serve hot.

GROUND LAMB WITH PEAS

***Preparation time**: 15 min*
***Cooking time:** 55 min*
***Portions:** 4*
Ingredients:
1 tbsp of coconut oil
3 dried red chillies
1 cinnamon stick (2 inches)
3 green cardamom pods
½ tsp of caraway seeds
1 medium red onion, chopped
1 piece of fresh ginger (¾ inch), chopped
4 cloves of garlic, minced
1½ tsp of ground coriander
½ tsp garam masala
½ tsp ground cumin
Ingredients:
½ tsp ground turmeric
¼ tsp ground nutmeg
2 bay leaves
1 pound lean ground lamb
½ cup Roma tomatoes, chopped
1-1½ cups of water
1 cup fresh green peas, shelled
2 tbsps plain Greek yoghurt, whipped
¼ cup fresh coriander, chopped
Salt and freshly ground black pepper, to taste

Directions:

In a Dutch oven, melt the coconut oil over medium-high heat. Add the red chillies, cinnamon stick, cardamom pods and cumin seeds and fry for about thirty seconds. Add the onion and fry for about 3-4 min.

Add the ginger, garlic cloves and spices and fry for about 30 seconds. Add the lamb and cook for about 5 min. Add the tomatoes and cook for about 10 min. Add the water and green peas and cook, covered, for about 25-30 min.

Add the yoghurt, coriander, salt and black pepper and cook for about 4-5 min. Serve hot.

ROAST LAMB CHOPS

Preparation time: *15 min*
Cooking time: *half an hour*
Portions: *4*
Ingredients:
For the lamb marinade:
4 cloves of garlic, minced
1 (2 inch) piece of fresh ginger, chopped
2 green chillies, seeded and chopped
1 tsp of fresh lime zest
2 tsp of garam masala
1 tsp ground coriander
1 tsp ground cumin

½ tsp ground cinnamon

1 tsp of coconut oil, melted

2 tbsps fresh lime juice

6-7 tbsps of plain Greek yoghurt

1 (8 bones) lamb chops, cut into pieces

Ingredients:

2 onions, sliced

For Relish:

½ garlic, chopped

1 (1 inch) piece of fresh ginger, chopped

¼ cup fresh coriander, chopped

¼ cup fresh mint, chopped

1 green chilli pepper, seeded and chopped

1 tsp of fresh lime zest

1 tsp organic honey

2 tbsps of fresh apple juice

2 tbsps fresh lime juice

Directions:

For the chops in a very mixer, add all the ingredients except the yoghurt, chops and onions and pulse until smooth. Transfer the mixture to a large bowl with the yogurt and stir to combine well. Add the chops and coat generously with the mixture. Place in the fridge to marinate for about twenty-four hours.

Preheat the oven to 375 degrees F. Line the baking tray with aluminium foil. Place the onion wedges in the bottom of the prepared baking dish. Arrange the rack of lamb on top of the onion wedges. Roast *for about half an hour. Meanwhile for the relish in the blender, add all the ingredients and pulse until smooth. Serve the chops and onions together with the relish.*

BAKED MEATBALLS WITH SHALLOTS

Preparation time: *20 min*
Cooking time: *35 min*
**Portions: 4-6*
Ingredients:
For the meatballs:
1 lemongrass stalk, outer peel peeled and chopped
1 (1½-inch) piece of fresh ginger, sliced -
3 cloves of garlic, minced
1 cup fresh coriander leaves, coarsely chopped
½ cup fresh basil leaves, coarsely chopped
2 tbsps plus 1 tsp fish sauce
2 tbsps of water
2 tbsps fresh lime juice
Ingredients:
½ pound lean minced pork meat
1 pound of lean minced lamb
1 carrot, peeled and grated
1 organic egg, bea10
For the shallots: -
16 shallot stalks, chopped
2 tbsps coconut oil, melted - Salt, to taste

½ cup of water

Directions:

Preheat oven to 375 degrees F. Grease a baking sheet. In a blender, add the lemongrass, ginger, garlic, fresh herbs, fish sauce, water and lime juice and blend until finely chopped.

Transfer the mixture to a bowl with the remaining ingredients and mix until well combined. Make 1-inch balls with the mixture.

Place the balls in the prepared baking tin in a single layer. In another rimmed baking tin, arrange the shallot stalks in a single layer. Drizzle with coconut oil and sprinkle with salt. Pour the water into the baking dish and cover 1 tightly with aluminium foil.

Cook the shallots for about half an hour. Cook the meatballs for about 30-35 min. Pork with peppers This dish not only tastes wonderful, but is also full of nutritional benefits.

PORK CHILLI

Preparation time: 15 min
Cooking time: 60 min
Portions: 8
Ingredients:
2 tbsps organic extra virgin olive oil
2 pounds of minced pork

1 medium red pepper, seeded and chopped

1 medium onion, chopped

5 cloves of garlic, finely chopped

1 part (2 inches) chilli, ground

1 tbsp ground cumin

1 tsp ground turmeric

Ingredients:

3 tbsps of chilli powder

½ tsp of chipotle chilli powder - Salt and freshly ground black pepper, to taste

1 cup of chicken broth

1 (28-ounce) may fire-roasted, crushed tomatoes

2 medium-sized bokchoy heads, sliced

1 avocado, peeled, pitted and chopped

Directions:

In a large frying pan, heat the oil over medium heat. Add the pork and fry for about 5 min. Add the pepper, onion, garlic, chilli and spices and fry for about 5 min. Add the stock and tomatoes and bring to the boil.

Add the bokchoy and cook, covered, for about twenty min. Uncover and cook for about twenty and a half hours. Serve hot with an avocado garnish.

PORK AND MUSHROOM MEATBALLS IN THE OVEN

Preparation time: *15 min*

Cooking time: 15 min
Portions: 6

Ingredients:
1 pound of lean pork
1 egg white,
4 fresh shiitake mushrooms, cut and chopped
1 tbsp fresh parsley, chopped
1 tbsp fresh basil leaves, chopped
Ingredients:
1 tbsp fresh mint leaves, chopped
2 tsp fresh lemon zest, finely grated
1½ tsp fresh ginger, finely grated
Salt and freshly ground black pepper, to taste

Directions:

Preheat the oven to 425 degrees F. Place the rack in the centre of the oven. Line a baking sheet with baking paper. In a large bowl, add all ingredients and mix until well combined.

Make equal-sized balls from the dough. Place the balls on the prepared baking tray in a single layer. Bake for about 12 quarters of an hour or until cooked through.

BEEF WITH CITRUS FRUIT AND BOK CHOY

Preparation time: 15 min
Cooking time: 11 min
Portions: 4

Ingredients:

For the marinade:

2 cloves of garlic, minced

1 (1 inch) piece of fresh ginger, grated

1/3 cup fresh orange juice

½ cup of coconut amino acids

2 tsp of fish sauce

2 tsp of Sriracha

1¼ pounds of sirloin steak, thinly sliced and trimmed

Ingredients:

For the vegetables:

2 tbsps of coconut oil, divided by

3-4 wide strips of fresh orange peel

1 jalapeño pepper, thinly sliced

½ pound of green beans, cut and halved crosswise

1 tbsp arrowroot powder

½ pound bokchoy, chopped

2 tsp of sesame seeds

Directions:

For the marinade in a large bowl, mix together garlic, ginger, orange juice, coconut aminos, fish sauce and Sriracha. Add the beef and coat generously with the marinade. Refrigerate to marinate for about a couple of hours. In a large frying pan, heat the oil over medium-high heat. Add the orange zest and fry about 2 min.

Remove the beef from the bowl, reserving the marinade. In the pan, add the beef and increase the heat to high.

Fry for about 2-3 min or until golden brown. Using a slotted spoon, transfer the beef and orange strips to a bowl. Using a paper towel, wipe the pan dry. In a similar skillet, heat the remaining oil over medium-high heat.

Add the jalapeño pepper and green beans and fry for about 3-4 min. Meanwhile, add the arrowroot powder to the reserved marinade and stir to combine. In the pan, add the marinade mixture, beef and bokchoy and cook for about 1-2 min. Serve hot with a garnish of sesame seeds.

MINCED BEEF WITH CABBAGE

Preparation time: 10 min
Cooking time: 15 min
Portions: 6
Ingredients:
1 tbsp olive oil
1 onion, thinly sliced
2 tsp fresh ginger, chopped
4 cloves of garlic, minced
1 pound lean ground beef
Ingredients:
1½ tbsps fish sauce
2 tbsps fresh lime juice
1 small head of purple cabbage, shredded
2 tbsps of peanut butter

½ cup fresh coriander, chopped

Directions:

In a large frying pan, heat the oil over medium heat. Add the onion, ginger and garlic and fry for about 4-5 min. Add the beef and cook for about 7-8 min, breaking it up with a spoon.

BEEF CHILI WITH VEGETABLES

Preparation time: 15 min
Cooking time: 1 hour
Portions: 6-8
Ingredients:
2 pounds lean ground beef
- ½ head of cauliflower, cut into large pieces
- 1 onion, chopped
- 6 cloves of garlic, minced
- 2 cups pumpkin puree
- 1 tsp dried oregano, crushed
- 1 tsp dried thyme, crushed
- 1 tsp ground cumin
- 1 tsp ground turmeric

Ingredients:
- 1-2 tsp of chilli powder
- 1 tsp of paprika
- 1 tsp cayenne pepper
- ¼ tsp red pepper flakes, crushed - Salt and freshly ground black pepper, to taste

- 1 (26-ounce) can tomatoes, drained
- ½ cup of water
- 1 cup of meat stock

Directions:

Heat a large frying pan over medium-high heat. Add the beef and fry for about 5 min. Add the cauliflower, onion and garlic and fry for about 5 min.

Add the spices and herbs and mix well. Reduce the heat to low and simmer, covered, for about 30-45 min. Serve hot.

BEEF MEATBALLS IN TOMATO SAUCE

Preparation time: 20 min
Cooking time: 37 min
Portions: 4

Ingredients:

For the meatballs:
- 1 pound lean ground beef
- 1 organic egg
- 1 tbsp fresh ginger, chopped
- 1 garlic oil, crushed
- 2 tbsps fresh coriander, finely chopped
- 2 tbsps of tomato paste
- 1/3 cup almond flour
- 1 tbsp ground cumin -

Pinch of ground cinnamon - Salt and freshly ground

black pepper, to taste
- ¼ *cup of coconut oil*

Ingredients:

For the tomato sauce:
- *2 tbsps of coconut oil*
- ½ *small onion, chopped*
- *2 cloves of garlic, minced*
- *1 tsp fresh lemon peel, finely grated*
- *2 cups of tomatoes, finely chopped*
- *Pinch of ground cinnamon*
- *1 tsp red pepper flakes, crushed*
- ¾ *cup of chicken broth - Salt and freshly ground black pepper, to taste*
- ¼ *cup fresh parsley, chopped*

Directions:

For the meatballs, in a large bowl, add all the ingredients except the oil and mix until well combined. Make balls of about 1 inch from the mixture. In a substantial skillet, melt the coconut oil over medium heat. Add the patties and cook for about 3-5 min or until golden brown on all sides.

Transfer the meatballs to a bowl. For the sauce, in a large frying pan, melt the coconut oil over medium heat. Add the onion and garlic and sauté about 4 min. Add the lemon zest and fry about 1 minute.

Add the tomatoes, cinnamon, red pepper flakes and stock and simmer for about 7 min. Add the salt, black pepper and meatballs and reduce the heat to medium-low. Simmer for about 20 min. Serve hot with all the parsley toppings.

SPICY LAMB CURRY

Preparation time: 15 min
Cooking time: 2 quarters of an hour
Portions: 6-8
Ingredients:
For the spice mixture:
- 4 tsp of ground coriander
- 4 tsp of ground cumin
- ¾ tsp of ground ginger
- 2 tsp ground cinnamon
- ½ tsp of ground cloves
- ½ tsp ground cardamom
- 2 tbsps sweet paprika
- ½ tsp of cayenne pepper
- 2 tsp of chilli powder
Ingredients:
- 2 tsp of salt
For Curry:
- 1 tbsp of coconut oil
- 2 pounds of boneless lamb, trimmed and cut into 1-inch cubes - Salt and freshly ground black pepper, to taste
- 2 cups onions, chopped

- 1¼ cup water
- 1 cup of coconut milk

Directions:

For the spice mixture in a bowl, mix together all the spices. Set aside. Season the lamb with salt and black pepper. In a large Dutch oven, heat the oil over medium-high heat. Add the lamb and sauté for about 5 min.

Add the onion and cook for about 4-5 min. Add the spice mixture and cook for about 1 minute. Add the water and coconut milk and bring to the boil over high heat. Reduce the heat to low and simmer, covered, for about 1-120 min or until the lamb is cooked to your desired doneness. Uncover and simmer for about 3-4 min. Serve hot.

GROUND LAMB WITH HARISSA

Preparation time: 15 min
Cooking time: 1 hour 11 min
Portions: 4

Ingredients:

1 tbsp extra virgin olive oil
- 2 red peppers, seeded and finely chopped
- 1 yellow onion, finely chopped
- 2 cloves of garlic, finely chopped
- 1 tsp ground cumin
- ½ tsp ground turmeric

Ingredients:
- ¼ tsp ground cinnamon
- ¼ tsp ground ginger
- 1 1/2 pounds lean ground lamb - Salt, to taste
- 1 can of diced tomatoes
- 2 tbsps harissa
- 1 cup water - Chopped fresh coriander, for garnish

Directions:

In a large frying pan, heat the oil over medium-high heat. Add the pepper, onion and garlic and fry for about 5 min. Add the spices and fry for about 1 minute. Add the lamb and salt and cook for about 5 min, breaking it up into pieces.

Add the tomatoes, harissa and water and bring to the boil. Reduce the heat to low and simmer, covered, for about 1 hour. Serve hot using the harissa garnish.

PAN-FRIED LAMB CHOPS

Preparation time: 10 min
Cooking time: 4-6 min
Portions: 4

Ingredients:
4 cloves of garlic, peeled - Salt, to taste
- 1 tsp black mustard seeds, finely crushed
- 2 tsp of ground cumin
- 1 tsp ground ginger

Ingredients:
- 1 tsp ground coriander
- ½ tsp ground cinnamon - Freshly ground black pepper, to taste.
- 1 tbsp of coconut oil
- 8 medium-sized lamb chops, sliced

Directions:

Place the garlic cloves on a cutting board and sprinkle with a little salt. With a knife, crush the garlic until it forms a paste. In a bowl, mix together the garlic paste and the spices.

Using a clear, crispy knife, make 3-4 cuts on both sides in the chops. Rub the chops generously with the garlic mixture. In a large frying pan, melt the butter over medium heat. Add the chops and cook for about 2-3 min per side or until desired doneness.

LAMB AND PINEAPPLE KEBAB

Preparation time: 15 min
Cooking time: 10 min
Portions: 4-6

Ingredients:
1 large pineapple, cut into 1½ inch cubes, split
- 1 piece of fresh ginger (½ inch), chopped
- 2 cloves of garlic, minced - Salt, to taste

Ingredients:

- Lamb shoulder steak 16 to 24 ounces, cut and diced 1½ inches -
Fresh mint leaves from a bunch
- Cinnamon powder, to taste

Directions:

In a blender, add about 1 1/2 servings of pineapple, the ginger, garlic and salt, and blend until smooth. Transfer the mixture to a large bowl. Add the chops and coat them generously with the mixture.

SPICED PORK ONE

Preparation time: 15 min
Cooking time: 60 min
Portions: 6

Ingredients:

1 (2 inch) piece of fresh ginger, chopped
- 5-10 cloves of garlic, minced
- 1 tsp ground cumin
- ½ tsp ground turmeric
1 tbsp ground hot paprika
- 1 tbsp red pepper flakes - Salt, to taste
- 2 tbsps apple cider vinegar
- 2 pounds pork shoulder, diced 1½ inches

Ingredients:
- 2 cups of domestic hot water, divided by
- 1 (1 inch wide) ball of tamarind pulp

- ¼ cup of olive oil
- 1 tsp black mustard seeds, crushed
- 4 green cardamoms
- 5 whole cloves
- 1 cinnamon stick (3 inches)
- 1 cup onion, finely chopped
- 1 large red pepper, seeded and chopped

Directions:

In a food processor, add the ginger, garlic, cumin, turmeric, paprika, red pepper flakes, salt and apple cider vinegar and pulse until smooth. Transfer the mixture to a large bowl. Add the pork and coat it generously with the mixture.

Set aside, covered for about an hour at room temperature. In a bowl, add 1 cup of hot water and the tamarind and set aside until the water cools. Using your hands, crush the tamarind to extract the pulp.

Add the remaining cup of hot water and stir until well combined. Through a fine sieve, strain the tamarind juice into a bowl. In a large frying pan, heat the oil over medium-high heat. Add the mustard seeds, green cardamoms, cloves and cinnamon stick and fry for about 4 min.

Add the onion and fry for about 5 min. Add the pork and fry for about 6 min. Add the tamarind juice and bring to the boil. Reduce the heat to medium-low and simmer for 1½ hours. Add the pepper and cook for about 7 min.

PORK CHOPS IN CREAMY SAUCE

Preparation time: 15 min
Cooking time: 14 min
Portions: 4

Ingredients:
2 cloves of garlic, minced
- 1 small jalapeño pepper, chopped
- ¼ cup of fresh coriander leaves
- 1½ tsp turmeric powder, separated
- 1 tbsp fish sauce
- 2 tbsps fresh lime juice

Ingredients:
- 1 can of coconut milk (13½-ounce)
- 4 pork chops (½ inch thick)
- Salt, to taste
- 1 tbsp of coconut oil
- 1 shallot, finely chopped

Directions:

In a blender, add the garlic, jalapeño pepper, cilantro, 1 tsp turmeric powder, fish sauce, lime juice and coconut milk and blend until smooth.

Sprinkle the pork evenly with the remaining salt and turmeric. In a frying pan, melt the butter over medium-high heat. Add the shallots and sauté for about 1 minute. Add the chops and cook for about 2 min per side. Transfer the chops to a bowl. Add the coconut mixture and bring to a boil.

Reduce the heat to medium and simmer, stirring occasionally, for about 5 min. Add the pork chops and cook for about 3-4 min. Serve hot.

DECENT BEEF AND ONION STEW

Preparation time: 10 min
Cooking time: 1-2 hours
Portions: 4

Ingredients:

2 pounds lean beef, cubed
3 pounds shallots, peeled
5 garlic cloves, peeled, whole
3 tbsps of tomato paste

Ingredients:

1 bay leaf
¼ cup of olive oil
3 tbsps of lemon juice

Directions:

Take a stew pot and put it on a medium heat. Add the olive oil and let it heat up. Add the meat and let it brown.

Add the remaining ingredients and cover with water. Bring everything to the boil. Reduce the heat to a minimum and cover the pot. Simmer for 1-2 hours until the meat is cooked through. Serve hot!

Chapter Five

SNACKS & DESSERTS

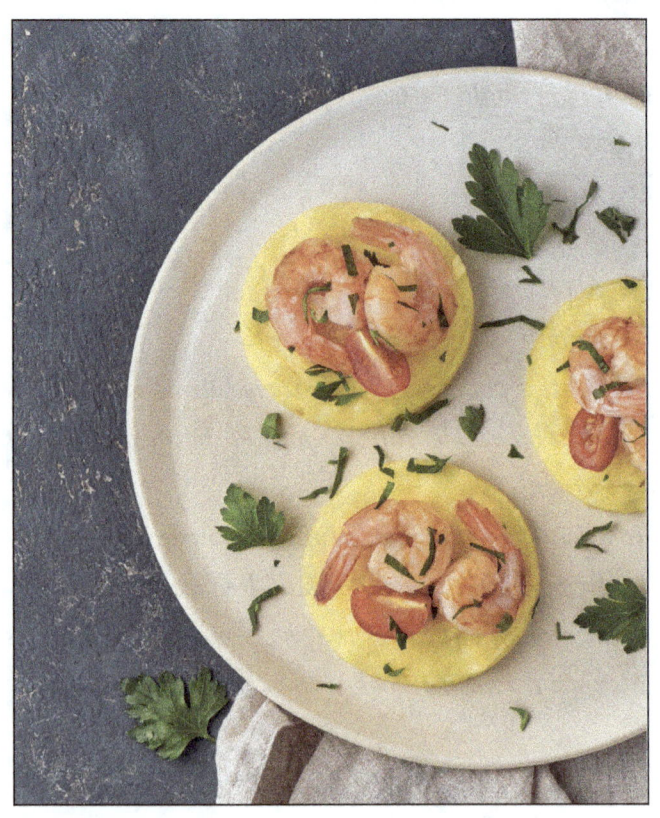

STRAWBERRY AND AVOCADO MIXTURE

Preparation time:
Cooking time: *5 min*
Portions: *4*
Ingredients:
2 cups of strawberries, cut in half
1 avocado, pitted and sliced
Ingredients:
2 tbsps chipped almonds
Directions:
Place all the ingredients in a bowl. Stir to combine. Leave to cool in the fridge before serving.

HONEY AND BERRY GRANITA

Preparation time: *10 min + freezing time*
Cooking time:
Portions: *4*
Ingredients:
1 tsp lemon juice
¼ cup of honey
1 cup fresh strawberries
Ingredients:
1 cup fresh raspberries
1 cup of fresh blueberries

Directions:

Bring 1 cup of water to the boil in a saucepan over high heat. Stir in honey until dissolved. Remove from heat and stir in berries and lemon juice; let cool.

Once cooled, add the mixture to a food processor and pulse until smooth. Transfer to a shallow glass and freeze for 1 hour. Stir with a fork and freeze for a further 30 min. Repeat a couple of times. Serve in dessert dishes.

CHOCOLATE-COVERED STRAWBERRIES

Preparation time: *15 min + cooling time*
Cooking time:
Portions: *4*

Ingredients:
1 cup of chocolate chips
¼ cup coconut flakes
1 pound of strawberries
Ingredients:
½ tsp of vanilla extract
½ tsp nutmeg powder
¼ tsp of salt
Directions:

Melt the chocolate chips for 30 seconds. Remove and stir in vanilla, nutmeg and salt. Leave to cool for

2-3 min. Dip the strawberries in the chocolate and then in the coconut chips.

Place on a biscuit sheet lined with greaseproof paper and leave for 30 min until the chocolate dries. Serve.

SUMMER FRUIT SORBET

Preparation time: *10 min + freezing time*
Cooking time:
Portions: *4*

Ingredients:

¼ cup of honey

4 cups of watermelon cubes

Ingredients:

¼ cup of lemon juice

12 mint leaves to serve

Directions:

In a food processor, blend the watermelon, honey and lemon juice to form a chunky puree. Transfer to a freezer-proof container and place in the freezer for 1 hour.

Remove the container and scrape with a fork. Place back in the freezer and repeat the process every half hour until the sorbet is completely frozen, about 4 hours. Distribute in bowls, garnish with mint leaves and serve.

HONEY PUDDING WITH KIWI

Preparation time:
Cooking time:
Portions:
Ingredients:
2 kiwis, halved and sliced
1 egg
2 ¼ cups of milk
Ingredients:
2 kiwis, halved and sliced
1 egg
2 ¼ cups of milk
Directions:
In a bowl, beat the egg with the honey. Stir in 2 cups of milk and vanilla. Pour into a saucepan over medium heat and bring to a boil. Combine cornstarch and remaining milk in a bowl.
Pour slowly into the saucepan and boil for 1 minute until thickened, stirring often. Divide between 4 cups and transfer to the fridge. Add the kiwis and serve.

PEACH CAKE WITH WALNUTS AND SULTANAS

Preparation time: 50 min + cooling time

Cooking time:
Portions: 6

Ingredients:

2 peaches, peeled and chopped

½ cup sultanas, soaked

1 cup plain flour

3 eggs

1 tbsp dark rum

¼ tsp cinnamon powder

1 tsp of vanilla extract

1 ½ tsp baking powder

Ingredients:

4 tbsps of Greek yoghurt

¼ cup of coconut oil

¼ cup of olive oil

2 tbsps of honey

1 cup of brown sugar

4 tbsps walnuts, chopped

¼ tsp caramel sauce

Directions:

Preheat oven to 350 °F. In a bowl, mix the flour, cardamom cinnamon, vanilla, baking powder and salt. In another bowl, beat the eggs with the Greek yogurt using an electric mixer. Gently add the coconut and olive oil. Combine well.

Add the rum, honey and sugar; stir to combine. Mix the wet ingredients with the dry mixture. Stir in the peaches, sultanas and nuts. Pour the mixture into a greased pan and bake for 30-40 min until a knife inserted into the centre of the cake comes out clean.

Remove from the oven and leave to rest for 10 min, then invert onto a wire rack to cool completely. Heat the caramel sauce in a pan and pour over the cooled cake to serve.

A HEARTY CHIA AND BLACKBERRY PUDDING

Preparation time: 45 min
Cooking time:
Portions: 2
Ingredients:
¼ cup chia seeds
½ cup blackberries, fresh
1 tsp liquid sweetener 1
Ingredients:
cup of coconut and almond milk, whole and unsweetened
1 tsp of vanilla extract
Directions:
Take the vanilla, liquid sweetener and almond milk and add to the blender. Process until thick. Add the blackberries and process until smooth.
Divide the mixture between cups and chill for 30 min. Serve and enjoy!

DELICATE BLACKBERRY CRUMBLE

Preparation time: *10 min*
Cooking time: *45 min*
Portions: *4*
Ingredients:
½ cup of coconut flour
½ cup banana, peeled and mashed
6 tbsps of water
3 cups of fresh blackberries
Ingredients:
½ cup arrowroot flour
1½ tsp of bicarbonate of soda
4 tbsps almond butter, melted
1 tbsp fresh lemon juice
Directions:
Preheat the oven to 300 degrees F. Take a baking tray and grease it lightly. Take a bowl and mix all the ingredients except the blackberries, mix well.
Place the blackberries on the bottom of the baking tray and cover with flour. Bake for 40 min. Serve and enjoy!

FANTASTIC MAPLE PECAN BACON SLICES

Preparation time: *10 min*

Cooking time: *25 min + freezing time*
Portions: *12*
Ingredients:
1 tbsp sugar-free maple syrup
12 slices of bacon
Granular stevia as desired
15-20 drops of Stevia
Ingredients:
For coating:
4 tbsps of dark cocoa powder
¼ cup pecans, chopped
15-20 drops of Stevia
Directions:
- Take a baking tray and lay the bacon slices on it. Rub with maple syrup and stevia, turn the slices over and do the same with the other side. Bake for 10-15 min at 220 degrees F. After cooking, drain the bacon fat.
- To form a batter, mix the bacon fat, stevia and cocoa powder. Dip the bacon slices in the batter and roll in the chopped pecans. Leave to air dry until the chocolate hardens.

CARROT BALL DELIGHT

Preparation time: *10 min*
Cooking time:

Portions: 4

Ingredients:

6 pitted Medjool dates

1 carrot, finely grated

¼ cup of raw walnuts

Ingredients:

¼ cup unsweetened coconut, shredded

1 tsp nutmeg

1/8 tsp sunflower seeds

Directions:

Take a food processor and add the dates, ¼ cup grated carrots, coconut sunflower seeds, nutmeg. Mix well and reduce the mixture to a puree.

Add the walnuts and the remaining ¼ cup of carrots. Pulse the mixture until it has a chunky consistency. Form small balls with your hand and roll them in the coconut. Cover with the carrots and cool. Enjoy!

FRIENDLY SPICE MUFFINS

Preparation time: 5 min
Cooking time: 45 min
Portions: 12

Ingredients:

½ cup raw hemp hearts

½ cup of linseed

¼ cup chia seeds

2 tbsps psyllium husk powder

Ingredients:

1 tbsp cinnamon stevia flavouring

½ tsp baking powder

½ tsp of sunflower seeds

1 cup of water

Directions:

Preheat the oven to 350 degrees F. Line the muffin tray with liners. Take a large bowl and add the peanut almond butter, pumpkin, sweetener, coconut almond milk, flax seeds and mix well. Continue stirring until the mixture is fully combined. Take another bowl and add the baking powder, spices and coconut flour. Mix well.

Add the dry ingredients to the wet bowl and stir until the coconut flour is well mixed in. Let sit for a while until the coconut flour has absorbed all the moisture.

Divide the mixture between your muffin tins and bake for 45 min. Enjoy your meal!

FANTASTIC CAULIFLOWER BAGELS

Preparation time: 10 min
Cooking time: 30 min
Portions: 12

Ingredients:

1 large cauliflower, topped and roughly chopped

¼ cup of nutritional yeast

¼ cup almond flour

½ tsp of garlic powder

Ingredients:

1 ½ tsp of fine sea sunflower seeds

1 whole egg

1 tbsp sesame seeds

Directions:

Preheat oven to 400 degrees F. Line a baking sheet with baking paper; set aside. Blend the cauliflower in a food processor and transfer to a bowl.

Add the nutritional yeast, almond flour, garlic powder and sunflower seeds to a bowl and mix. Take another bowl and beat the eggs, add them to the cauliflower mixture. Give the mixture a stir. Incorporate the mixture into the egg mixture.

Make balls with the dough, making a hole in each ball with your thumb. Place them on the prepared sheet, flattening them into the shape of a bagel. Sprinkle with sesame seeds and bake for 30 min. Remove from the oven and leave to cool, enjoy!

LIME PIE

Preparation time: *5 min*

Cooking time: *5 min + freezing time*

Portions: *12*

Ingredients:

1 tbsp ground cinnamon

3 tbsps almond butter

1 cup of almond flour

For the filling:

3 tbsps of grass-fed almond butter

Ingredients:

4 ounces of whole cream cheese

¼ cup of coconut oil

2 files

A handful of baby spinach Stevia to taste

Directions:

Mix the cinnamon and almond butter to form a crumble mixture. Press this mixture into the bottom of 12 muffin cups. Bake for 7 min at 350 degrees F.

Squeeze the lime and grate the zest while the crust is cooking. Take a food processor and add all the filling ingredients. Blend until smooth. Leave to cool naturally. Pour the mixture into the centre. Freeze until ready to serve.

THE PERFECT PONZU ORANGE

Preparation time: *30 min*

Cooking time: *5 min*

Portions: *8*

Ingredients:

¼ cup coconut amino acids

½ cup rice vinegar

2 tbsps of dried fish flakes

Ingredients:

1 (1 inch) square of kombu (kelp)

1 orange, cut into four

Directions:

Take a saucepan and place it over a medium heat. Add the coconut amino acid, rice vinegar, fish flakes, kombu and orange quarters and leave the mixture to stand for 30 min.

Bring the mixture to the boil and remove from the heat immediately. Allow to cool and strain through cheesecloth. Serve and enjoy!

THE REFRESHING NUTTER

Preparation time: *10 min*
Cooking time:
Portions: *1*

Ingredients:

1 tbsp chia seeds

2 cups water 1 ounce macadamia nuts

Ingredients:

1-2 packets of stevia, optional

1 ounce hazelnuts

Directions:

Add all the listed ingredients to a blender. Blend on high speed until smooth and creamy. Enjoy your smoothie.

APPLE AND ALMOND MUFFINS

Preparation time: 10 min
Cooking time: 20 min
Servings: 6 muffins

Ingredients:

6 ounces of ground almonds

1 tsp cinnamon

½ tsp baking powder

1 pinch of sunflower seeds

Ingredients:

1 whole egg

1 tsp apple cider vinegar

2 tbsps erythritol

1/3 cup apple juice

Directions:

Preheat oven to 350 degrees F. Line a muffin pan with paper cups; set aside. Mix the almonds, cinnamon, baking powder and sunflower seeds together and set aside. Take another bowl and whisk the eggs, apple cider vinegar, apple sauce and erythritol.

Add the mixture to the dry ingredients and mix well until a smooth batter is obtained. Pour the batter *into the mould and bake for 20 min. Once done, leave to cool. Serve and enjoy!*

MATCHA BOMB SUPREME

Preparation time: *100 min*
Cooking time:
Portions: *10*
Ingredients:
3/4 cup hemp seeds
½ cup of coconut oil
2 tbsps of coconut almond butter
1 tsp Matcha powder
Ingredients:
2 tbsps vanilla pod extract
½ tsp of mint extract
Liquid stevia
Directions:
Take your blender/food processor and add the hemp seeds, coconut oil, Matcha, vanilla extract and stevia.
Mix until you have a nice batter and divide into silicone moulds. Melt the coconut and almond butter and pour over the top. Let the cups cool and enjoy!

PINEAPPLE HEART PUDDING

Preparation time: 10 min
Cooking time: 5 hours
Portions: 4

Ingredients:
1 tsp baking powder
1 cup of coconut flour
3 tbsps of stevia
3 tbsps avocado oil
½ cup of coconut milk
Ingredients:
½ cup pecans, chopped
½ cup pineapple, chopped
½ cup lemon peel, grated
1 cup pineapple juice, natural
Directions:

Grease the slow cooker with oil. Take a bowl and mix the flour, stevia, baking powder, oil, milk, pecans, pineapple, lemon zest, pineapple juice and stir well.

Pour the mixture into the slow cooker. Put the lid on and cook on LOW for 5 hours. Divide between bowls and serve. Enjoy!

TASTY POACHED APPLES

Preparation time: *10 min*
Cooking time: *2 hours 30 min*
Portions: *8*
Ingredients:
6 apples, core, peel and slices
1 cup apple juice, natural
Ingredients:
1 cup of coconut sugar
1 tbsp cinnamon powder
Directions:
Grease the slow cooker with cooking spray. Add the apples, sugar, juice and cinnamon to the slow cooker. Stir gently.
Put the lid on and cook on HIGH for 4 hours. Serve cold and enjoy!

HEART-WARMING CINNAMON RICE PUDDING

Preparation time: *10 min*
Cooking time: *5 hours*
Portions: *4*
Ingredients:
6 ½ cups of water
1 cup of coconut sugar
2 cups of white rice

Ingredients:

2 cinnamon sticks

½ cup coconut, shredded

Directions:

Add the water, rice, sugar, cinnamon and coconut to your Slow Cooker. Stir gently. Put the lid on and cook on HIGH for 5 hours. Discard the cinnamon.

Divide the pudding between dessert plates and enjoy!

Chapter Six
CONCLUSIONS

Dash Diet is easy to follow and readily available food guide recipes for people who want to lose weight to improve their health. It is designed to lower blood pressure and help you lose weight without the need to count calories. This cookbook has no limitations on food portions. However, it is essential to make the right choices. The dash diet follows a healthy approach. It aims to help you enjoy a long life.

Anyone who wants to lose weight can eat on the dash diet. This diet limits the intake of salt, fats, and oils. The dash diet is not vegetarian. However, vegetarians can still use this diet. They should avoid dairy products and avoid the use of animal fats. Vegetarians who eat fish should avoid salt and animal fats. The dash diet is very flexible. It shows you how to make great-tasting food that you and your family can enjoy.

The primary purpose is to help people who have low self-esteem to improve their health and daily life. You will see the benefits to your health if you follow this diet, maintain glucose metabolism, and avoid obesity.

Exercise and diet changes can help you reduce weight and control blood pressure. In addition, keeping track of your performance with exercise or physical activity can help you maintain motivation for a more extended period. Similarly, a diet record is also helpful in estimating your daily intake and calories consumed per day.

The Dash strategy is a new way of eating - for living. So when you stray from the eating plan for a few days, don't let that stop you from reaching your health goals.

Ask yourself why you got off track.

Get back on track. Here's how: Tell yourself why you got off the path. Was it the drinking at a party? Did you experience tension at home or work? Find out what started your detour, and then start the Dash plan again. Figure out if you tried to do too many things at once. Anyone starting a new lifestyle sometimes tries to change too much at once. Instead, one or two things should be changed at a time. The only way to succeed is, slowly but surely. Break the process down into small steps. This not only deters you from doing too many things at once, but it also makes the changes easier. Break complicated goals into smaller, more manageable steps, each attainable. Keep a log of what you eat and what you do. This can help you understand the problem. The record also allows you to make sure each food group and physical activity is sufficient each day. You will see many changes in your lifestyle. Your meals, blood pressure, and health will improve. This will help you live better, and you will be healthier.

www.ingramcontent.com/pod-product-compliance
Lightning Source LLC
Chambersburg PA
CBHW070920080526
44589CB00013B/1375